Rowan Hillson, MD, FRCP is a Consultant Physician with a special interest in Diabetes at The Hillingdon Hospital, Middlesex. She wrote her first books about diabetes while working in Oxford where she completed several diabetes research projects. Now she shares the care of several thousand people with diabetes with other members of the Hillingdon Diabetes Team. Dr Hillson is an enthusiast of outdoor activities and she takes groups of diabetics of all ages on Outward Bound courses. She works closely with the British Diabetic Association, and has a particular interest in helping people with diabetes to learn more about their condition.

GW00600776

The British Diabetic Association is pleased to be able to recommend this book as a useful guide for those who already have a general understanding of diabetes and how to manage it, but now want further guidance.

For those wanting more basic or general information the BDA recommends Dr Rowan Hillson's *Diabetes: The Complete Guide*. For a complete list of recommended BDA publications please telephone 0800 585088 or contact their Careline on 0171 636 6112.

THE BRITISH DIABETIC ASSOCIATION

The BDA has been helping people with diabetes for over 60 years. Since it was set up in 1934 by RD Lawrence and the author HG Wells, both of whom had diabetes, the BDA has concentrated on care and research.

The BDA has a very active branch network with over 450 branches nationwide. These include specialist groups for young people, parents and Asian people. In June 1994, they opened their first regional office in Glasgow and they now have offices in Warrington, Walsall and Belfast. A further six are planned across the UK. Regional offices aim to help improve the provision of health care through the NHS at local level, support the local Area Co-ordinators and Branches, and provide information and a presence on a regional basis.

The BDA is dedicated to fighting prejudice and the myths that surround diabetes. They do this by increasing awareness of the condition through advertising and the media. They also work to influence government policy, act as the voice of diabetes and campaign for the best care, the best quality of life, an end to unfair discrimination, and much more.

The BDA's Careline offers help and support on all aspects of diabetes. It provides a confidential service which takes general enquiries from people with diabetes, their carers and from health care professionals. The specialist staff can give you the latest information on topics such as taking care of your diabetes, diet information and information on children with diabetes, their parents and families.

The BDA is one of the largest funders of diabetes research in the UK. If you would like to contact the British Diabetic Association or become a member, you can telephone on 0171 323 1531 between 9am and 5pm Monday to Friday or write to them at 10 Queen Anne Street, London, W1M 0BD.

LATE ONSET
DIABETES

*A practical guide to
managing diabetes over 40*

Dr Rowan Hillson
MD FRCP

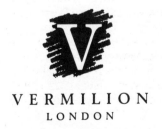

VERMILION
LONDON

For Kay and Rodney Hillson, and Marjorie Lee.

Copyright © Rowan Hillson 1988, 1996

1 3 5 7 9 10 8 6 4 2

First edition published by Macdonald Optima in 1988 as
Diabetes Beyond 40

This revised, second edition published in the United Kingdom in
1996 by Vermilion an imprint of Ebury Press

Random House UK Ltd
Random House
20 Vauxhall Bridge Road
London SW1V 2SA

Random House Australia (Pty) Ltd
20 Alfred Street, Milsons Point, Sydney,
New South Wales 2016, Australia

Random House New Zealand Limited
18 Poland Road, Glenfield,
Auckland 10, New Zealand

Random House, South Africa (Pty) Limited
Box 2263, Rosebank 2121, South Africa

Random House UK Limited Reg. No. 954009

A CIP catalogue record for this book is available from the British
Library.

ISBN 0 09 181406 5

Typeset in Palatino by Deltatype, Ellesmere Port
Printed and bound in Great Britain by Mackays of Chatham, plc

Papers used by Vermilion are natural, recyclable products made
from wood grown in sustainable forests.

CONTENTS

ACKNOWLEDGMENTS

I wrote this book for my patients and it is they who taught me much of its contents. I thank all the over-forties with diabetes whom I have met through the years for sharing so much with me.

This book would not have been written without the support of my parents, Mr and Mrs W.R. Hillson, and my brother and his wife, Dr and Mrs S.W. Hillson, and I greatly appreciate their unfailing encouragement.

I am extremely grateful to all my colleagues in Oxford for their help and for giving me so much of their very valuable time. In particular I would like to thank Dr T.D.R. Hockaday and Dr J.L. Mann for their comments. I also thank Oxford Regional Health Authority.

I would also like to thank the following people for their permission to use some of the material reproduced in this book: The *Journal of the Royal College of Physicians of London* for the table shown on page 25 taken from volume 17, no. 1 of January 1983; MIMS for the table of insulins on page 59, for the table of blood glucose testing strips and meters on page 71 and for the table of finger prickers and compatible lancets on page 71. (These charts are updated monthly in MIMS.); and to Synergist Ltd for permission to use the illustration on page 131.

Thanks are also due to Maggie Raynor and Peter Cox for the line drawings and to Harriet Griffey and Philippa Stewart for their constant enthusiasm. Photographs by R. Hillson.

INTRODUCTION

This book is for people with diabetes who are over forty years old. This does not mean that the under-forties are not allowed to read it! Much of the information in this book applies to *all* adults with diabetes. I have tried to write a book which will not only help someone with newly-diagnosed diabetes understand and learn to care for their condition, but will also extend and update diabetes knowledge in those of you who have had diabetes for many years.

New discoveries are being made in the diabetes research laboratories throughout the world. Over recent years the treatment of diabetes has become more effective and easier to manage. It is important for people with diabetes to take full advantage of advances in knowledge. Sometimes, while knowledge is developing, there may be different views about how a particular aspect of diabetes should be treated. I have tried to present the generally-accepted view, but please remember that there are hundreds of thousands of people with diabetes, every one of you different, and thousands of doctors treating diabetes, all with slightly different ideas on treatment. Your particular version of diabetes may need treatment which differs from that described here. Please discuss your treatment with your doctor – he or she will help you in the way that you personally need.

I believe that people with diabetes should enjoy life to the full and that it is possible for most of you to do what you want at work and during your leisure time. I also believe that it is the individual himself or herself who should manage his or her diabetes, with help from the professionals whenever it is needed. At first you will need a lot of help but gradually you will gain in confidence in diabetes self-care, although you will always need regular check-ups. If you are going to rule your diabetes you need to learn as much as you can about the condition in general and how it affects you in particular. I hope that this book will help you to do this.

1

A person with diabetes

This is a book for the people on the receiving end – those with diabetes and their carers – so I am going to start at the beginning from the patient's point of view and not with a textbook summary of the disease. However, I shall use the correct medical terms as they arise so that you will know what they mean if your doctor uses them. There is also a glossary on page 167.

How can untreated diabetes make its presence felt?

No symptoms at all

Some people discover that they have diabetes when they attend an insurance medical or routine health check. Even in retrospect they may have felt they had no symptoms, although most people, when they feel the benefits of treatment, realise that they were not 100 per cent fit before diagnosis. In an Oxford study one in eight people with newly-diagnosed maturity-onset type diabetes had no symptoms at all.

Feeling off-colour (malaise)

We all have off days, but untreated diabetes may make you feel vaguely unwell for most of the time. You may find your job gradually becomes more tiring. You may be snappy or irritable or find decisions harder to make. Life may not be such fun any more.

Lack of energy

The walk to work may seem longer and your muscles more tired after exercise. Sports and active hobbies may suffer as your physical performance declines, or you may have to make a much greater effort to achieve previously-easy physical goals.

Thirst, drinking large volumes of fluids (polydipsia) and passing large volumes of urine (polyuria)

Unlike the common but non-specific symptoms I have just described, these symptoms are relatively specific for diabetes. Two in three people with newly diagnosed maturity-onset diabetes are thirsty. The thirst is such that you need to drink literally pints of fluids, both during the day and through the night. You may have a persistently dry mouth and sometimes a nasty taste on your tongue. You may have to start carrying cans of drinks around with you.

The need to pass large volumes of urine frequently can be embarrassing. You may have to get up several times each night to urinate. Men may notice that they have small white sugar spots on their shoes if urine has splashed there and dried and, in tropical countries, ants may gather around urine passed by someone with untreated diabetes.

Weight loss

Although many people with untreated diabetes feel generally unwell, it does not usually suppress the appetite. Indeed, you may actually have a craving to eat more, especially sweet foods. However, even if you are eating more than usual, you may start to lose weight. The ancient Greeks believed that in diabetes flesh was melted down and passed out in the urine – a supposition not far from the truth. Initially you may lose fatty tissue (which may please those who are overweight and have been trying to slim); then, if the condition remains untreated, you may see loss of muscle bulk as well.

Tingling, pins and needles (paraesthesia)

We have all experienced tingling when our leg has 'gone to sleep' if we have put pressure on it for a long time. People with diabetes may feel this in their hands and feet, even if they have not pressed on them.

Visual changes

Some people find that they have diabetes when they visit an eye specialist – maybe because their vision is blurred or their usual glasses no longer seem to be satisfactory. There may be problems in focusing. Do not buy new spectacles or contact lenses until your diabetes has been treated for several weeks – you may no longer need them, as such changes in focusing are temporary.

Itching

Sometimes people with diabetes may have generalised itching. More often this is localised between the legs, due to fungal infection (see below).

Infections

If you have untreated diabetes you may be plagued by boils or other skin infections, which recur after treatment. Women are often diagnosed as having diabetes when they go to their family practitioner or gynaecologist with soreness and itching between the legs (pruritus vulvae), usually due to the fungal infection thrush (moniliasis). Cystitis or urinary tract infection is also common in women with untreated diabetes. Men may develop thrush on the penis (balanitis) and urinary infections too. Other infections such as pneumonia may take longer to resolve in someone with unrecognised diabetes, especially in older people.

Constipation

Because your body is becoming dry you may find that your motions become drier and harder to pass and that you open your bowels less frequently.

Cramp

People with diabetes seem more prone to cramp in the legs and other parts of the body than non-diabetics.

Questions the doctor will probably ask you

About yourself as a person

Your doctor will want to know your age and about your job, sports or hobbies, as these will all influence your treatment. He or she will try to find out a little about 'what makes you tick'. He will also ask about your worries and for your ideas about what you feel is wrong with you. When he has made a full assessment, this will all help him to explain to you what is going on and give you the most appropriate advice.

Family history

Do you have relatives at home that you have to care for and support? A family history of diabetes makes it more likely that you will have diabetes than if you have no diabetic relatives. Other conditions that run in families, like thyroid disease and pernicious anaemia, may be associated with a tendency to diabetes.

Pregnancy

Women who have had big babies or who had diabetes while they were pregnant are likely to develop diabetes in later life.

Other illnesses

If you have a hormone disorder such as thyroid disease, or rarer conditions such as Cushing's syndrome (steroid excess), you may have a tendency to diabetes. Alternatively, your diabetes may be making an existing illness worse.

Medication

Some drugs can bring a tendency to diabetes out into the open, such as water tablets (diuretics); others may cause diabetes, such as steroid drugs. Other drugs which you take may affect the way in which your diabetes is managed.

Signs of untreated diabetes

Nothing abnormal

Most new diabetics have nothing abnormal to find on examination.

General lack of vitality

This may be noted in the way people move and respond.

Weight loss

This is often obvious in someone with new diabetes.

Fluid depletion

Someone with severe polyuria may be very fluid-depleted and may have dry skin, mouth and tongue.

Pulses

Some people with diabetes have hardened arteries (atherosclerosis) and may have poor circulation, with cold hands and feet.

Blood pressure

Many people with diabetes, especially if they are overweight, have high blood pressure (hypertension). If you are very fluid-depleted your blood pressure will be low and may fall when you stand, making you feel dizzy (postural hypotension).

Eyes

People with new diabetes sometimes have cataracts in the lens of their eyes which disappear when the diabetes is controlled. Longer-term cataracts and problems with the circulation to the retina at the back of the eye may also occur in diabetes.

Sensation

Diabetes can impair the function nerves which sense touch, pin-pricks, heat, cold and vibration, so your doctor will test these.

Allergies

If you are allergic to sulphonamide drugs you may be allergic to medication prescribed for diabetes. It is always important for any doctor you see to know about all your drug allergies.

Smoking

This is dangerous, whether you have diabetes or not.

Diet, including alcohol intake

Both your calorie intake and the sorts of foods which you eat will be assessed by your doctor or dietitian. Eating and drinking a lot of sugary foods may have helped worsen your diabetes. If further assessment confirms diabetes you will need appropriate dietary advice to fit in with your energy needs and meal arrangements.

What now?

If you have some of the symptoms described above, with or without any abnormalities on examination, your doctor will suspect that you have diabetes. Now he has to prove the diagnosis.

Urine test

The oldest and simplest method of detecting diabetes is to test your urine for glucose. If it is present it almost always indicates diabetes.

In previous centuries the doctor used to taste the urine! Nowadays a chemically-impregnated stick is dipped into your urine and an answer is available in a minute or less. The presence of glucose in the urine is called glycosuria. However, a urine test should not be used as the sole evidence on which to base a diagnosis of diabetes.

Blood tests

Glucose is a simple sugar derived from sugary or starchy foods. Most people have between 4 and 7.8 millimoles (mmol) of glucose in each litre of their blood (or 72 to 140 milligrams (mg) per decilitre for American readers). To diagnose diabetes you must have more than 11.0 mmol/l

(200 mg/dl) of glucose in your blood. One reading like this in someone with symptoms of diabetes is sufficient to confirm the diagnosis. A blood glucose level which is higher than normal is called hyperglycaemia (hyper = high, glycaemia = blood glucose).

If your doctor wants to be sure in a borderline case he may ask you to come back another day after fasting, and measure your blood glucose before and after a glucose drink. If you have had nothing to eat since midnight the night before, your whole blood glucose should be below 7.8 mmol/l (140 mg/dl). Levels above this suggest that you may have diabetes.

It is easier to diagnose diabetes than it is to prove that someone is not diabetic. If your blood glucose level (random or fasting) is below 5.5 mmol/l (100mg/dl) it is extremely unlikely that you have diabetes. Blood glucose levels vary considerably following food. If your blood glucose level is between 5.5 (100 mg/dl) and 7.8 mmo/l (140 mg/dl) fasting, or 5.5 (100 mg/dl) and 11.1 mmol/l (200 mg/dl) after eating, your doctor may request a glucose tolerance test. This involves attending the laboratory having had nothing but plain water to drink since midnight. A blood glucose sample will be taken, then you will be given a drink containing 75 grammes (g) glucose. Two hours later another blood glucose test is taken (some laboratories do tests in between).

The results of the glucose tolerance test are interpreted as follows:

Blood glucose concentration (venous plasma sample)	
Fasting below 7.8 mmol/l (140 gm/dl)	Normal
Two hour below 7.8 mmol/l (140 mg/dl)	
Fasting below 7.8 mmol/l (140mg/dl)	Impaired glucose
Two hour between 7.8 and 11.1 mmol/l (200 mg/dl)	tolerance
Fasting above 7.8 mmol/l (140 mg/dl)	Diabetes
Two hour above 11.0 mmol/l (200 mg/dl)	

Summary

- Symptoms of uncontrolled diabetes are feeling vaguely unwell, lack of energy, thirst, drinking a lot of fluid, passing a lot of urine, weight loss, pins and needles, blurred vision, itching, infection, constipation and cramps. Many people have no symptoms at all.
- Most people with newly-diagnosed diabetes have no clinical signs unless their blood glucose is very high or they have had untreated diabetes for a long time.
- If you have glucose in your urine you probably have diabetes.
- If your blood glucose level is above 11.0 mmol/l (200 mg/dl) and you have any of the symptoms described above you definitely have diabetes.

2

What is diabetes?

Definition of diabetes mellitus

Diabetes mellitus is a condition in which the blood glucose concentration is higher than normal. The condition was named by the Greeks – diabetes means siphon, reflecting the polyuria, and mellitus means sweet like honey, reflecting the glucose in the urine. Two out of every 100 people in the West have diabetes. The older people become, the more likely they are to have or develop diabetes. Between four to ten out of every 100 people over sixty have diabetes. However we think that only one out of every two people with diabetes knows they are diabetic.

Impaired glucose tolerance or chemical diabetes

For many years there has been dispute about which levels of blood glucose to take as defining normality and which to take as defining diabetes. The World Health Organisation has now identified a grey area in which the blood glucose is above normal but not high enough to mean that a person is obviously diabetic. This lies between 7.8 and 11.1 mmol/l (140 and 200 mg/dl) after food, and is called impaired glucose tolerance (see page 8).

Impaired glucose tolerance is a state in which the body cannot cope with glucose efficiently. This state may return to normal, remain unchanged or progress to diabetes. People with impaired glucose tolerance are at greater risk of heart and circulatory problems than those with normal glucose tolerance. If you have impaired glucose tolerance follow a diabetic diet, maintain a desirable weight for your height and exercise regularly (after discussion with your medical adviser).

'False' diabetes

Some people show glucose in the urine more easily than others. The amount of glucose in the urine is determined by the kidneys. Under normal circumstances, i.e. with the blood glucose between 4 and 7.8 mmol/l (72 and 140 mg/dl), no glucose escapes into the urine. However, as the glucose levels rise above this, more and more glucose enters the urine.

The blood glucose level at which glucose starts to appear in the urine, the threshold, varies from person to person. It is usually around 10 mmol/l (180 mg/dl). The higher the kidney threshold, the higher the blood glucose at which urine glucose tests become positive. However, if the threshold is lower than usual someone with a normal blood glucose may have glycosuria. This is called renal (kidney) glycosuria and may lead to a false diagnosis of diabetes. This is why we always measure the blood glucose, if necessary after a standard glucose drink by mouth, before labelling anyone as diabetic.

Diabetes insipidus

This is a rare condition caused by deficiency of the water-retaining hormone called anti-diuretic hormone, due to brain or pituitary gland disease. Symptoms are thirst, polyuria, polydipsia and weight loss but there is *no* glucose in the urine (diabetes = siphon, insipidus = tasteless). It is nothing to do with diabetes mellitus.

This book is about diabetes mellitus. This is rather long winded, so from now on I will refer to it simply as diabetes.

Why is the blood glucose raised?

Normal glucose metabolism

To answer this question we first need to consider normal glucose metabolism. Metabolism is the chemical processing of substances in the body. Starchy or sugary foods are broken down into simple sugars, e.g. glucose, fructose and lactose. These simple sugars are absorbed into the bloodstream from the gut and pass through the liver into the rest of the body. Glucose is the body's main energy source, although energy can be made from other sugars and by breaking down fats and proteins. The brain's sole energy source is glucose.

Before glucose can be used it has to enter the body's cells. It cannot do this without insulin, which inserts itself into places on the outside of the cell called receptors. This sends a signal to the cell to activate glucose transporters to carry the glucose inside and to start using it. The receptor is like a keyhole in a door in the cell wall and insulin is the key which opens the door for glucose to enter. Once in the cell the glucose is either used to produce energy straightaway or converted into a storage compound called glycogen.

Insulin

This hormone or chemical messenger is made in tiny clusters of cells known as islets of Langerhans in the pancreas. The pancreas is a gland which lies behind the stomach, at the back of the abdominal cavity. Insulin is stored in these islet cells and released when the blood glucose level rises. There is always a small amount of circulating insulin, but this level is increased by ten times or more after a meal.

Insulin acts mainly on the liver, muscles and fatty tissues.

The liver

In the last century diabetes was thought to be a liver disease. This is partly true. In the presence of insulin, liver cells take up glucose from the bloodstream and store it as glycogen. If there is too little insulin the liver cannot store glucose but releases huge quantities into the bloodstream. This is the main reason why a person with untreated diabetes has a high blood glucose. Insulin lack also allows proteins to be broken down into glucose.

The muscles

Muscles need insulin to take up and store glucose so that it can be used to make energy. If there is no insulin when you

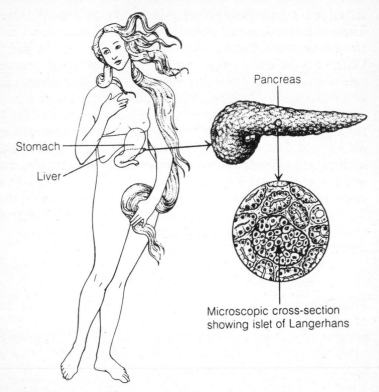

Pancreas

Stomach

Liver

Microscopic cross-section
showing islet of Langerhans

*Position of liver and pancreas, with detail showing insulin-
producing islet cells in pancreas.*

exercise, muscles cannot take up more glucose when their
stores are used up.

Fatty tissue

Fat cells need insulin to take up the breakdown products of
digested fat from the bloodstream and store them for future
use. Without insulin the fat stores start to break down into
fatty acids, which are then released into the bloodstream.

Insulin – an allrounder

If you have diabetes you do not make enough insulin, and
without insulin glucose cannot be stored or used for energy.
Glucose from food stays in the bloodstream and the liver
releases more glucose from its stores; body fat breaks down

into fatty acids, and proteins break down into glucose. Glucose builds up in the bloodstream and pours out in the urine. You lose weight.

Different types of diabetes

So far it may seem straightforward – diabetes is due to insulin deficiency. However when it became possible to measure blood insulin levels accurately two broad groups of results were found. Some people indeed had no insulin in their blood; most of them were young and thin. But some had very high insulin levels in their blood; most of these were over thirty and overweight. And they all had diabetes. What was going on?

The answer would seem to lie in the insulin receptors and the chemical signals that are triggered when insulin links with the receptor. Recent research has shown that some families with diabetes inherit specific defects in the way in which their insulin receptors signal to the cell. These people became resistant to the action of insulin. It is as if the key fits the keyhole but cannot turn the lock and the glucose cannot enter the cell. As yet, these very specific inherited signalling defects have been found in only a small proportion of people with diabetes. However, it appears that receptor problems are common. For example, insulin receptors seem to work less efficiently in people who are overweight. More and more insulin is required to overcome the problem. The high concentrations of insulin may themselves further reduce the efficiency of the receptor system.

Insulin production may be inefficient – for example, insulin may be released too early or too late to cope with a meal, or the natural rhythm of insulin production may be disturbed. In some people insulin production gradually fails – this can be particularly problematic in people who need a lot of insulin to overcome insulin resistance.

Over the years there have been heated discussions about the classification of diabetes. It is now clear that there are many different causes of diabetes, all with the same end result – unduly high blood glucose levels. At present diabetes

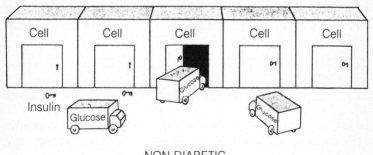

NON-DIABETIC

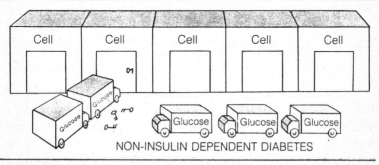

NON-INSULIN DEPENDENT DIABETES

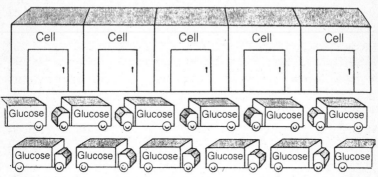

INSULIN-DEPENDENT DIABETES

Simplified diagrams showing insulin, insulin receptors and the uptake of glucose by cells in the different types of diabetes.

is divided into two main types – insulin-dependent diabetes mellitus (IDDM) and non-insulin-dependent diabetes mellitus (NIDDM).

Insulin-dependent diabetes mellitus (IDDM)

This is also called *juvenile-onset diabetes* or *Type I* diabetes. IDDM classically affects people under 30 years of age, including children. It is associated with an absence of insulin; onset may be abrupt, with severe symptoms. The only treatment is insulin injections. It occurs in one person in 400.

Non-insulin-dependent diabetes mellitus (NIDDM)

This is also called *maturity-onset diabetes* or Type II diabetes. NIDDM usually affects older people, who are often, but not always overweight. Blood insulin concentrations may be high to start with and can ultimately fall. It is in this group that there seems to be problems with insulin receptors and their signalling systems. NIDDM is probably a mixture of many different causes of diabetes. It is usually gradual in onset and symptoms may develop insidiously. Initially, NIDDM may be treated by diet, especially weight reduction, with or without glucose-lowering pills. Insulin injections are usually not needed, although eventually they may be necessary in some people with NIDDM. It is for this reason that the term 'non-insulin-dependent' is disliked by some authorities as being imprecise.

Why did you get diabetes?

In some families, precise genetic defects in receptor-signalling systems have been identified (see page 14). If one identical twin has this form of diabetes the other will nearly always develop it eventually . If you have NIDDM, some 25 per cent of your first-degree relatives (that is parents, sisters, brothers or your children) have or will develop diabetes. If both you and your partner have NIDDM, there may be a three in four chance that your child will eventually develop diabetes. The risk is about one in seven if one parent has diabetes.

IDDM is linked with specific genetic markers. If you have these you are more likely to have diabetes than people without these markers. If two insulin-dependent diabetics marry, there may be a one in four chance that their child will have diabetes. One in seventeen children of IDDM fathers develops diabetes. The risk is one in 100 if the mother has IDDM.

Other factors

The body has protective mechanisms which attack foreign material such as bacteria. Sometimes the body attacks its own cells by mistake. Insulin-producing cells can be destroyed in this way. Virus infections may be a trigger of this reaction.

Summary

- Diabetes mellitus is a condition in which the blood glucose is higher than normal.
- The elevation of blood glucose is due to insulin lack. Insulin acts on insulin receptors on cells, mainly in the liver, fatty tissue and muscles.
- Insulin deficiency may be absolute, because the pancreas is not making it, or relative, because the insulin that is made does not link with enough insulin receptors to act on the cells.
- IDDM diabetes is associated with absolute insulin deficiency. It usually occurs in young people, giving severe symptoms. Insulin treatment is essential.
- NIDDM diabetes is usually associated with relative insulin deficiency. It tends to occur in older people who are overweight and symptoms may be gradual in onset. This type of diabetes may respond to diet alone or to pills.
- Some people have forms of diabetes which do not fit clearly into any type. Their diabetes can be treated as well as that of people with more clearly-defined types of diabetes.

3

Looking after your diabetes

Now you know that you have diabetes and you know what diabetes is. But what is it going to mean to you? Is it going to interfere with your well-being? Is it going to stop you doing things? Is it going to interfere with your job? Upset your family? Is it ever going to go away? What is going to happen to you?

The first point is that once you have been diagnosed diabetic, you need to accept your condition and look forward to sorting it out. And note that I said *you* need to sort it out. Diabetes is not a condition like appendicitis, in which the surgeon removes your appendix for you while you just lie there anaesthetised. Diabetes is a condition in which the person who has it is the single most important factor in determining the outcome.

This does not mean that you are on your own – far from it. Your diabetes care team are always there to guide and support you in whatever way you need. But remember that you are the most important member of the team looking after your diabetes.

What you need to know right now is what you have to do over the next few days to start getting yourself better and preventing any further deterioration in your condition. You will gradually learn more and more about diabetes and how to care for it.

Share your feelings

First, share your grief, anger, frustration and worry with someone you trust who is a good listener. Try not to bottle it all up.

I can reduce some of your worries straightaway by telling you that properly cared-for diabetes will not reduce your well-being. It will not stop you doing things and is unlikely to interfere with your job. Obviously your family will be upset at first because they care for you; they will be sad and angry and frustrated too. But sharing the early worries with your family helps. Diabetes will not stop you from taking your usual part in family life and from keeping your family responsibilities. Diabetes is for ever, but many people with maturity-onset diabetes can control their blood glucose with a diabetic diet and by keeping to their ideal body weight.

What is going to happen to you? Fear of the unknown is always worrying. In this book I will explain about diabetes and its effects on the body and how to cope with it. If you know what is going on you can learn to manage it.

Beginners' diet

I will tell you in detail about your diet in the next chapter – you may be surprised to find that a diabetic diet is virtually the same as the healthy diet recommended for everyone nowadays. At present the following simple rules will help your body:

- Remember that your body cannot deal with sudden glucose loads. If glucose is absorbed gradually you will be able to metabolise it more easily.
- Stop eating very sweet things like sweets, candy, chocolates, cakes, biscuits, puddings and fizzy drinks.
- Do not put sugar in tea or coffee. If you need a sweet taste use artificial sweeteners in moderation – there is a wide range to choose from.
- Introduce more high-fibre foods like vegetables, wholewheat bread, beans, bran.
- Cut down on very fatty foods like cream, butter, margarine and fried foods.
- If you are overweight, eat a little less of everything, especially fats.

- If you are thirsty have low-calorie drinks or water. Tea and coffee are all right with artificial sweeteners and preferably skimmed or semi-skimmed milk.

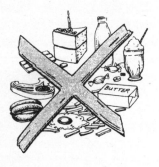 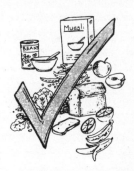

Cut down on sweet and fatty foods and introduce more high-fibre foods.

Treatment

If the doctor gives you pills for your diabetes, write down their name, dose and exactly when he wants you to take them, i.e. before, with or after meals and which meals. Then take them as instructed.

These pills will be to lower your blood glucose. Occasionally people are very sensitive to them and the blood glucose falls lower than expected. This is called hypoglycaemia and is rare but if you feel unwell or odd in any way, eat some sugar or something sweet and contact your doctor.

Finding out what is happening – urine testing

Ignorance is not bliss! Learn how to check your own blood glucose, then you will not have to wait for your doctor to tell you how you are getting on.

An indirect method of doing this is by measuring how much glucose has overflowed into the urine. A non-diabetic has none and that is what you should be aiming at.

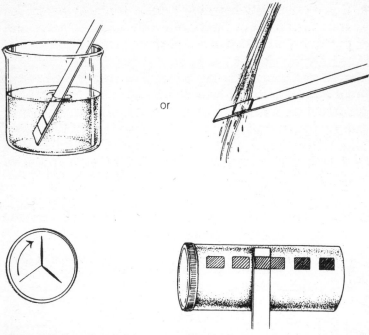

Urine testing dip-sticks.

Nowadays there are simple dip-sticks with which to check urine glucose, e.g. Chemstrips uG, Clinistix, Diastix, Diabur 5000, Medi-Test. Your doctor can give them to you on prescription or you can buy them at any chemist or drug store. Read the instructions carefully.

All these sticks have a felt-like pad at one end. Hold the stick so that the pad is in the stream of urine (or pass urine into a clean container and dip the pad into it), tap off the excess urine, wait the length of time stated in the instructions, usually one minute, and match the colour of the pad against the colour code provided by the manufacturers. At this stage what you need to know is if there is no glucose in the urine (good), some, e.g. less than 1 per cent (fair), a lot, i.e. 1 per cent or more (not so good). If you have some or a lot and it does not decrease over the next week, your treatment needs adjusting, so contact your doctor.

If you prefer you can learn how to check your blood glucose on finger prick samples (see Chapter 8).

The next steps

Hopefully this chapter has given you enough information to survive and to start feeling better. The rest of the book is about returning to full health and taking full command of your diabetes and its management. The first cornerstone of diabetes management is finding out what is going on in your body (information), the second the correct diet, the third exercise and the fourth drug treatment. All of these will be considered individually.

Summary

- Start accepting your diabetes. Share your feelings.
- Cut out very sweet, sugary and very fatty foods. Eat more fibre. If you are fat, eat a little less of everything.
- Take any pills prescribed by your doctor. Write down his instructions and learn the name of your pills.
- Learn how to test your urine for glucose so that you can check on what is happening.

4

Diet

A diet is what you eat. It can be completely random or follow a planned pattern. In a planned diet there are two major factors to consider:

- How much you eat
- What you eat

People with diabetes need to consider both factors. The diabetic diet is the single most important part of the treatment of a person with diabetes.

How much you eat

You need to eat to stay alive. Why? Food is the body's fuel. Food is broken down to provide energy to keep essential body maintenance processes ticking over (like the heart beat and breathing, for example) and to power the muscles when you want to move. If you eat more than you need for that day's maintenance and muscle activities the body stores the excess as fat. If you eat less than you need on a particular day your body supplies 'internal food' by breaking down fat stores. Children and teenagers need additional food energy to help them to grow. If you are over forty you no longer need to eat to grow. Unless your job is very energetic physically you need to eat much less than you did as a teenager.

Energy taken in as food should balance energy used. If you eat just what you need each day you will stay the same weight. If you eat more than you need you will get fat. If you eat less than you need you will lose weight. Energy is measured in kilocalories, shortened to calories or kcals. It can also be measured in kilojoules. It helps if you have a general idea of approximately how much energy you use and how much energy different types of food contain.

Energy used

Body maintenance uses roughly 1000 to 2000 kcals a day, depending how much you weigh, on all sorts of other factors like how hot or cold the weather is, and individual factors such as your body build and your personal body chemistry. You would have to be very big to need as much as 2000 kcal a day just to keep the body ticking over. Activities also use variable amounts of energy – it depends how much effort you put into them and how efficient you are at doing an activity, as well as your size.

You use far fewer calories exercising than most people think. For example an hour's ironing by a medium-sized woman may use about 120 kcal. Similarly, you have to be a very active sportsman to expend a lot of calories in a single exercise session. If the same woman runs for an hour cross-country she might use 580 kcals. This 580 kcals can then be replaced by just 112 g (4 oz) of chocolate. But if you exercise regularly, say every day, you will gradually use up calories.

Acceptable weight

Studies, mainly by life insurance companies, have produced ranges of acceptable average weights for a given sex and height. Some people call these ideal body weights. But how do insurance companies work them out? By looking at the weight and height of men and women who die sooner than expected and those who live an average lifespan. The table shows acceptable average weights for men and women. What should you weigh?

16 Stone = .160
64
224 lb

Guidelines for body weight

Metric

Height without shoes (m)	Men Weight without clothes (kg)			Women Weight without clothes (kg)		
	Acceptable average	Acceptable weight range	Obese	Acceptable average	Acceptable weight range	Obese
1.45				46.0	42–53	64
1.48				46.5	42–54	65
1.50				47.0	43–55	66
1.52				48.5	44–57	68
1.54				49.5	44–58	70
1.56				50.4	45–58	70
1.58	55.8	51–64	77	51.3	46–59	71
1.60	57.6	52–65	78	52.6	48–61	73
1.62	58.6	53–66	79	54.0	49–62	74
1.64	59.6	54–67	80	55.4	50–64	77
1.66	60.6	55–69	83	56.8	51–65	78
1.68	61.7	56–71	85	58.1	52–66	79
1.70	63.5	58–73	88	60.0	53–67	80
1.72	65.0	59–74	89	61.3	55–69	83
1.74	66.5	60–75	90	62.6	56–70	84
1.76	68.0	62–77	92	64.0	58–72	86
1.78	69.4	64–79	95	65.3	59–74	89
1.80	71.0	65–80	96			
1.82	72.6	66–82	98			
1.84	74.2	67–84	101			
1.86	75.8	69–86	103			
1.88	77.6	71–88	106			
1.90	79.3	73–90	108			
1.92	81.0	75–93	112			

Non-metric

Height without shoes (ft, in)	Men Weight without clothes (lb)			Women Weight without clothes (lb)		
	Acceptable average	Acceptable weight range	Obese	Acceptable average	Acceptable weight range	Obese
4 10				102	92–119	143
4 11				104	94–122	146
5 0				107	96–125	150
5 1				110	99–128	152
5 2	123	112–141	169	113	102–131	154
5 3	127	115–144	173	116	105–134	161
5 4	130	118–148	178	120	108–138	166
5 5	133	121–152	182	123	111–142	170
5 6	136	124–156	187	128	114–146	175
5 7	140	128–161	193	132	118–150	180
5 8	145	132–166	199	136	122–154	185
5 9	149	136–170	204	140	126–158	190
5 10	153	140–174	209	144	130–163	196
5 11	158	144–179	215	148	134–168	202
6 0	162	148–184	221	152	138–173	208
6 1	166	152–189	227			
6 2	171	156–194	233			
6 3	176	160–199	239			
6 4	181	164–204	245			

Losing weight

Most of my readers will have NIDDM and most of you will
be overweight. How do you lose weight? Simple – take in less
energy than you use each day. By now some of you will be
yawning. Everyone knows that is how to lose weight. Why
labour the point? Well, just take a look around you next time
you come to a diabetic clinic. Everybody knows how to lose
weight but it is still very difficult for many people to put their
knowledge into practice. Why? We are not sure why some
overweight people have such difficulty in losing weight even
when they are eating very low-calorie diets. It seems that
some people's bodies are very good at storing food away and
not so good at using it up to make energy. But even for them
the basic principle holds true. If you take in less energy than
you use, you will eventually lose weight. More often it is our
lack of willpower which prevents us from losing weight.
Eating is fun and, for many people, eating lots is lots more
fun. So keep yourself occupied and do not give yourself time
to think about the food you must not eat. And always
remember the energy equations:

- Energy in equals energy out   . . . your weight stays
                                                           the same
- Energy in less than energy out . . . you lose weight
- Energy in exceeds energy out . . . you gain weight

Practicalities

So, am I saying that you have to measure the calorie count of
every single thing you eat if you want keep in energy
balance? No, of course not! Life is much too interesting to
waste time weighing all your food. But there are some simple
things you can do right away to control your calorie intake.

Reduce total quantity

If you are overweight, a simple reduction in every portion of
food you eat will go a long way to helping you lose weight.
Instead of having two spoonfuls, have one and a half. When

you spread margarine on your bread, scrape a little off again. Use small plates so that the portions look more. Eat with a small spoon or fork and put your knife, fork or spoon down between each mouthful. If you are full, leave the excess on your plate or put it away for another meal.

Improve your knowledge

Reducing all portions of food a little can help you to control your intake, but knowledge of how fattening different types of food are can make your diet more interesting and successful. We all have a fair idea of this already; what you need to do is build on this knowledge. For example:

- Very high calories, very fattening – Cream cakes, Butterscotch ice cream sundae with cream.
- Moderate calories, moderately fattening – Boiled chicken breast, Baked potato.
- Few calories, not fattening – Watermelon, Celery, Lettuce.
- No calories, not fattening at all – Water.

What you eat

We can progress some way towards energy balance without a detailed knowledge of dietetics or nutrition. However, to care for your diabetes properly, and to ensure that you not only remain in energy balance but in *healthy* energy balance, you need to know a little more about what kind of foods to eat.

What are foods made of?

Foods are combinations of carbohydrates (sweet foods like sugar, candy, jam, jelly, molasses, sweet biscuits, and starchy foods like bread, beans, lentils, potatoes, pasta, rice), proteins (e.g. meat, fish, soya), fats (e.g. cream, margarine, olive oil, lard), minerals, trace elements, vitamins and water. A good mixed diet will give you enough vitamins and trace elements, so I will not discuss these further.

Fats are very high-energy foods, containing 9 kcal/gram. Proteins and carbohydrate are medium-energy foods; they contain 4 kcal/gram. So a small slice of wholemeal bread would give about 40 kcal, but the pat of butter which you spread on it also provides 40 kcal. Cutting down on fatty foods will therefore help you to lose weight.

Carbohydrates

Within each type of food there are some that are better for people with diabetes than others. Remember that your body is not very good at coping with a sudden glucose load. Very sugary foods like candy or sweets are quickly broken down into simple sugars like glucose by digestive juices and absorbed fast. Your body cannot release a burst of insulin to cope with this glucose load, but it may be able to deal with a more gradual rise in glucose. So reduce your intake of sweets, chocolates, sweet cakes, sweet biscuits, jam and other sugary foods. If you must eat sugar, have it mixed in with a meal and not on its own. If you are on oral hypoglycaemic pills or insulin only eat sugary foods to treat a low blood glucose (see page 72) or to cover vigorous exercise (see page 37). Do not eat them at all if you are on diet treatment only. Try to re-educate your palate to like less sweet foods.

If you cannot manage tea or coffee without sugar use an artificial sweetener like saccharine or aspartame.

What carbohydrate foods are good for people with diabetes?

The answer is foods that release their simple sugars (mainly glucose) slowly during the digestion progress. These are foods which are high in fibre (which also makes the food more bulky and filling). The best sort of fibre is the type found in beans, peas and lentils, although fibre or roughage is also found in wholemeal bread, bran, whole-grain cereals and jacket potatoes. Other high-fibre foods are vegetables – cabbage and celery, for example.

What proportion of your diet should consist of carbohydrates?

Current recommendations are 50–60 per cent of daily calories. This is quite a lot of carbohydrate.

If you are taking pills to lower the blood glucose or insulin it is sensible to divide the carbohydrate foods out through the meals of the day. Snacks in between may also be helpful for insulin-treated people, but only as part of the total daily calorie intake. This is because the pills or insulin act throughout the day and, for practical purposes, most of their impact is upon glucose. A steady amount of glucose being absorbed from your food for your pills or insulin to act on will help you to obtain smoother control.

If you take insulin you should have three meals a day – breakfast, lunch and dinner – and three snacks – mid-morning, mid-afternoon and before bed. How much you eat at each time depends on your activity pattern, but a rough guide would be a quarter of your carbohydrate intake for each of the three main meals and the remaining quarter divided into snacks. If you are not taking insulin injections you will probably not need to eat snacks.

Portions, exchanges and the glycaemic index

In some clinics people with diabetes are taught an exchange system for carbohydrate foods (in America some clinics also teach protein and fat exchanges). This is based on the concept that 10 grams of carbohydrate from, say, bread, spaghetti and potato behaves the same way once swallowed no matter which food it came from. However nutritionists have pointed out that the amount by which 10 grams of one carbohydrate food, for example potato, raises the blood glucose is not necessarily the same as the blood glucose rise after 10 grams of carbohydrate in the form of spaghetti. The degree of blood glucose rise produced by a particular carbohydrate food is called the glycaemic index. Researchers continue to investigate this. Many factors determine how much glucose actually enters the bloodstream – how the food is cooked, what other foods it is mixed with, how much liquid is taken with it, and so on. Blood flow in your gut wall, stomach emptying rate, bowel transit time and other factors in your body may also influence the rate of absorption of a meal. Although it is imprecise some people find the carbohydrate exchange system helpful in balancing their diet, particularly if they are taking insulin.

What should you do?

Follow the system advised by your diabetic clinic and ask as many questions as you need to make sure that you have understood. It is helpful to know roughly how much carbohydrate there is in different starchy foods. If you wish, you can find out what effect different foods have on your blood glucose by measuring it two hours after a meal and noting the results. But please do not become obsessional about this – I found one woman testing all her drinks with her urine glucose strips to see if they were too sugary! That is going a little too far. If your diet seems very boring, unpalatable or incomprehensible discuss it again with the dietitian – it may be that you have not fully understood.

Bill and Myra were in their mid-seventies when Bill developed diabetes. They both listened carefully to the enthusiastic young dietitian as she explained about Bill's diet. She wrote it all down for them and they took the diet sheet home to study carefully. They puzzled and puzzled over it. For every meal Bill was supposed to eat a strange food called CHO. Neither of them could remember what the dietitian had said about CHO but it was obviously important. So Myra set out with her shopping bag to buy some. She tried two supermarkets and in each a helpful assistant searched along the shelves – no CHOs. She tried a delicatessen and two pharmacies. Finally a pharmacist explained that CHO was simply an abbreviation for carbohydrate!

Guar

Guar is a viscous fibre carbohydrate substance concentrated from cluster beans. Some doctors prescribe it as a way of adding fibre to the diet for people who might otherwise find it difficult to eat enough fibre. It is in the form of granules which can be mixed with water or juice and drunk immediately or sprinkled dry on food. In some studies large doses of guar have been shown to reduce the rise in blood glucose which occurs after each meal. Guar should be introduced very gradually and you must drink plenty of fluids to reduce the likelihood of indigestion, flatulence and diarrhoea.

'Diabetic foods'

A large choice of foods labelled 'diabetic' is available. There is no need to buy these. Most have replaced glucose or sugar with fructose or sorbitol. Very little is known about their metabolic effects. Taken in excess, sorbitol produces a rumbling stomach and diarrhoea. Fructose is as fattening as other carbohydrates, so fructose-containing foods should be eaten in small amounts only – it may be better to eat a little real chocolate or jam (jelly) with a meal than to use a lot of sorbitol. Nowadays there are plenty of high-fruit, reduced-sugar jams (jellies) available.

Low-calorie 'diabetic foods' which can be used are those in which sugar and glucose have been replaced by artificial sweeteners. Examples are diet Coca Cola and diet Pepsi Cola.

Protein

Proteins are the building blocks that the body needs to repair old cells and to manufacture new ones. You *must* eat sufficient protein; protein-containing foods like meat, fish, milk, cheese and eggs are an essential part of your diet. One of the problems of protein foods is that they frequently contain a lot of fat mixed in with the protein, this being especially true of dairy products and red meats.

Protein foods which are good for people with diabetes are chicken, turkey, white fish, skimmed milk and cottage cheese. Protein foods which should be eaten in small amounts only are beef and pork (cut all the extra fat off), hard cheese and oily fish. Two or three eggs a week is a reasonable number. If you are vegetarian you must remember to eat low-fat dairy produce regularly and include other sources of protein such as soya, quorn and nuts – peanuts have a high protein (and fat) content.

Fats

Amount

We all need a small amount of fat, but most of us eat far too much of it. Learn to watch the amount of fat in your diet and to cut it down as much as possible. Never eat unnecessary fat. Trim the fat off meat. Grill foods rather than fry them. Avoid crisps and potato chips or fries and eat your potatoes boiled in their skins or baked in their jackets. Use skimmed milk and keep cream as a very special treat. Use only low-fat salad dressings. Scrape your margarine on to bread or crackers.

Type

The type of fat you eat is important too. There is some evidence that saturated animal fats (dairy produce and fat on meat) are linked with heart and artery disease. Many doctors believe that polyunsaturated plant fats such as sunflower oil and margarine appear safer. You must remember, though, that saturated and polyunsaturated margarines have the same calorie content – so spread them thinly. Include mono saturates such as olive oil. There is still controversy about the effects of different types of fat on the development of heart and blood vessel disease, so ask your own doctor what he or she thinks.

Salt

It has been suggested that a high salt (sodium chloride) intake is associated with high blood pressure. Many doctors believe that this is so, although there is still some discussion about it. Recent research has suggested that the rise in blood glucose after eating starchy foods is greater if they are eaten with salt than if salt is not added.

The food that you eat contains more than enough salt for your body's daily needs. It therefore seems sensible not to add even more salt at the table. Train your palate to savour the subtle taste of the food itself without all the excess salt.

Alcohol

Can people with diabetes drink alcohol? Yes, in moderation. Three units of alcohol a day, e.g. one-and-a-half pints of beer, three *small* shorts, is reasonable. However, there are two things you have to remember. The first is that alcohol is a source of calories – it is very fattening. If you drink you should include the alcohol in your diet plan as a high-energy food. Beers and lagers and sweet wines or liqueurs have carbohydrate in them as well, but beware carbohydrate-reduced beers – the carbohydrate is reduced by brewing it further and making the beer more alcoholic.

The second problem is that alcohol stops the release of glucose from the liver. This may mean that if you take oral hypoglycaemic pills or insulin you may be at risk of a low blood glucose, or hypoglycaemia, when you drink alcohol. So never drink on an empty stomach.

Help

This may all sound very complicated if you are not used to thinking about your diet. Don't panic! The key to success is gradual adjustment until your diabetic diet is one which not only fulfils the requirements I have outlined but also suits your habits and lifestyle. Nothing terrible will happen if you make dietary mistakes. It is no good giving someone who is unused to high-fibre food a very high-fibre diet on day one. He will not eat it, or if he does he may get indigestion. But gradually replacing his white bread with wholemeal, slice by slice, using bran cereal mixed in with his cornflakes, adding a

few beans to the casserole, will help him to change in a
practical way.

The details

I have outlined the general principles of a diabetic diet. I have
not given diet sheets. At first it is more important to get the
overall idea than to grapple with the finer details. There are
several excellent books available which will help you to work
out your diet more precisely. Contact the British Diabetic
Association for a current list of recommended publications.

Summary

- Consider how much you eat.
- Remember the energy equation:
  Energy in equals energy out . . .
      your weight stays the same
  Energy in less than energy out . . .
      you lose weight
  Energy in exceeds energy out . . .
      you gain weight
- Learn which foods are very fattening, which less
  fattening.
- Adjust the amount you eat to your needs so that you
  achieve your ideal body weight and stay there.
- Consider what you eat.
- Your diet should contain 50–60 per cent carbohydrate,
  the rest as protein and fats.
- Starchy high-fibre carbohydrate foods are best. Sugary,
  refined carbohydrates are absorbed too fast for your
  body to cope with.
- Eat protein foods that have little fat in them.
- Reduce your total fat intake as much as possible.

- Eat polyunsaturated fats in preference to saturated ones.
- Avoid excess salt.
- And enjoy your food!

5

Exercise and relaxation

Everyone needs exercise to keep them fit and healthy. It makes you feel good and keeps you looking good. And in diabetes it helps with the energy balance equation. Excess weight will be lost more easily with regular exercise. Regular vigorous exercise keeps your heart healthy and promotes the circulation in your legs. It also increases insulin sensitivity by increasing the number and/or availability of insulin receptors on the cells. Exercise also keeps your body supple. But above all, exercise is fun. Two other books will help you to enjoy exercise to the full – *Diabetes: A Beyond Basics Guide* by Rowan Hillson and *The Diabetics' Get Fit Book* by Jackie Winter and Dr Barbara Boucher.

Glucose, insulin and exercise

Glucose from the food you eat is stored in the liver and muscles as glycogen. This storage process needs insulin. When you exercise, the glycogen in the muscles is broken down into glucose and used as energy. If more glucose is needed the muscles take it up from the bloodstream with the help of a little insulin. As the blood glucose levels fall the liver releases more glucose from its stores to top them up. This cannot happen in the presence of high insulin concentrations. Thus you can see that for exercise you need good glycogen stores in the muscle and a little insulin. Too much insulin will cause hypoglycaemia because the liver cannot top up the blood glucose from its stores. Too little insulin will cause a high blood glucose level and make exercise difficult because the muscles cannot take up glucose from the bloodstream.

Too little food before exercise will also cause hypoglycaemia. For all but very brief exercise you need a good supply of glucose in the blood. Some of this will come from the liver, the rest directly from food. High fibre foods provide steady amounts of glucose over several hours; sugary foods provide rapidly absorbed peaks of glucose to be used in vigorous exercise. If you exercise regularly your muscles will need less insulin to top up their glucose supplies and your insulin or oral hypoglycaemic dose may fall.

Check your blood glucose (see Chapter 8) before and after exercise to start with and at intervals thereafter to learn how much food and insulin or pills you need. If you are doing unaccustomed exercise you may need to reduce your insulin or pills and increase your food before the exercise period. You need some high-fibre carbohydrate a couple of hours before exercise in order to provide gradually-absorbed glucose and some rapidly-absorbed glucose immediately before and during exercise. Overweight people on diet alone do *not* need to eat extra! You will gradually be able to refine your treatment as your training programme progresses.

Andy is a marathon runner with diabetes. When he started training he reduced his insulin and ate more before running. Now running is part of his everyday life and so he does not need to adjust his insulin for running. He knows that one standard-sized Mars bar will last him for 10 miles. Most of us would need a lot more than a Mars bar to keep us going.

Getting fit

Athletes spend years training. No one expects them to win a gold medal in their first race. Similarly everyone has to accustom his or her body gradually to exercise. As we grow older our joints stiffen and our exercise capacity falls. An unfit teenager can get away with a sudden burst of energy, but an unfit seventy-five year old cannot – indeed his heart may be so startled by the sudden demands placed upon it that he has a heart attack. And he may be stiff and aching for days afterwards.

Start training gently. There are several aspects to training. You need to improve your breathing and circulation. You need to strengthen your muscles – particularly those most used in whichever activity you have chosen. You need to increase your suppleness. Your stamina must be extended gradually.

Wear comfortable clothes and shoes (training shoes which do not chafe anywhere are good) so that you can forget what you are wearing. You should be able to take a layer off as you warm up. Start with warming-up exercises for the whole body and finish with some cooling-down exercises, the amount of warming-up and cooling-down needed will depend on the type of activity pursued.

Warming up

- Stand upright and take some deep breaths, filling the whole of the lungs and emptying them completely.
- Gently stretch each part of the arms and legs, trunk and neck. Never do anything that hurts – pain is the warning signal that damage is about to be done. Stretch and relax each part several times.
- Then do a few flexing and extending exercises, say five repetitions of each. Go over each part of the body in turn.
- Then do something a little more vigorous, running on the spot, step-ups, bicycling on a machine if you have one. Start with less than five minutes and gradually extend the time.
- Now you are ready for your exercise.

Cooling down

- Repeat your flexing and extending exercises.
- Stand upright and take some deep breaths, filling the whole of the lungs and emptying them completely.
- Feel your muscles relax and all the tension flow away.
- Find somewhere warm and out of a draught to lie flat and undisturbed. Carry on breathing deeply but slowly (if you start feeling tingly or giddy you are overbreathing). Close your eyes. Relax completely.

- Have a glucose-containing drink, replacing fluid and energy.
- Have a shower, but comfortably warm not too hot.

What sort of exercise?

The important point about exercise is that it should be fun. Why spend time doing something you do not enjoy? It is easier to exercise in company but you may wish to start getting fit at home first. Do not be shy. Most of us are less fit than we would like to be. And few of us look slender and glamorous in a leotard or tracksuit. Choose an activity close to home if possible – you will be more likely to keep it up. Discuss your exercise plans with your doctor. Aim for just five minutes a day at first. You need to exercise at least three times a week to derive maximum benefit. However, aim for gentle progression and not exercise to exhaustion. Vigorous exercise should be tried only after at least a month of regular progressive gentle exercise and on the guidance of your doctor.

Walking

This is a form of exercise nearly everyone can do. It is free and can be adjusted to each person's level of fitness. You need comfortable shoes and waterproof and windproof clothing or something to shade you from over-hot sun, depending on climate. A folding umbrella is useful. Take a snack with you.

Start by thinking before each journey 'Do I really need to use the car?' If not, walk. Use the stairs and not the elevator – at least for a few floors. Do you really need to have everything delivered? My mother walks to the newsagent's to buy the paper every morning and enjoys looking at the gardens through the seasons. Have fun exploring your neighbourhood, looking at the shops. Go with a companion if you do not want to be alone. Walk in daylight and in safe neighbourhoods.

You may prefer to walk in the country; explore woodland

trails, country lanes. Gradually extend the distance and difficulty – more hills, more rough ground as you become fitter.

Gardening

Gardening can be as energetic as you make it – raking uses a lot of energy, while weeding can provide gentle exercise. Digging uses about six times the energy expended by someone sitting quietly. A short spell working in the garden every day will keep you fit and give you something beautiful to look at.

Exercise in the house

You do not need special equipment to exercise at home. One woman I know used to keep fit by running up and down her stairs twenty times a day. *The Diabetics' Get Fit Book* by Jackie Winter and Dr Barbara Boucher gives a complete home workout.

Swimming

This is another good form of exercise for all ages. It uses muscles throughout the body and can be varied according to your fitness level. The water helps to support you. If you do not know how to swim take lessons.

Choose a warm supervised pool with an end in which you can stand easily and steps in and out unless you are a good swimmer. Warm up before you start swimming. Have a meal an hour or two before swimming and eat some rapidly-absorbed carbohydrate immediately before entering the water. Carry glucose in a pocket in your swimming costume (Hypostop or Glutose gell in its polythene screwtop bottle are excellent). Swimming uses about seven times the energy expended while sitting relaxing. Never go swimming alone.

Sea swimming is also fun, but more hazardous. Use safe public beaches and obey warning notices. Remember that you can quickly get out of your depth and it is very tiring swimming against a current. Always swim with a friend and preferably on beaches supervised by a life guard. Beware of cramp when you are swimming and do not allow yourself to become chilled. If you are prone to cramp, quinine-containing drinks like slimline tonic or bitter lemon may help. After your swim dry yourself thoroughly and have something to eat.

Jogging and running

Over recent years jogging and running have become very popular. However there has also been a steady rise in jogging injuries. Do not be tempted to run before you can walk. Running or jogging on hard city streets places a considerable strain on your joints (which act as shock absorbers). You should build up to it slowly and gently, allowing your body to become used to these new demands. Do not go jogging simply because it is fashionable.

If you do decide that you would like to do jogging, choose your running shoes carefully (ask a senior assistant in a reputable sports shop or your chiropodist or podiatrist). Eat a light high-glucose snack before you start and carry glucose and your diabetic card with you. Do your warm-up exercises first. Run or jog a little further each day – and do not forget that you have to be able to get home as well. Running moderately fast needs about ten times the energy used when sitting down.

Aerobics

This is another popular way of keeping fit. The name really means nothing – nearly all forms of exercise are aerobic (i.e. need oxygen), unless continued for a very brief time like sprinting. What most people understand by aerobics is repetitive vigorous movements, usually to music, which produce shortness of breath and a marked increase in heart rate. It is a companionable pastime and usually gives most major muscles a workout. Take it gently and gradually increase; your teacher should ensure that you do this.

Aerobics uses eight or nine times the energy needed by someone sitting quietly.

Dancing

Some people prefer ballroom dancing, others more modern varieties. Remember not to drink too much alcohol, though – it reduces the amount of glucose released by the liver and you may need that glucose to dance with. Stick to soft drinks if you can, and either way eat something. Ballroom dancing uses about three times as much energy as sitting down, energetic modern dancing about the same as aerobics.

Squash and tennis

These are played in many countries and it is usually possible to get a game in any major city or town. Both, as with other forms of exercise, need building up to gradually.

Squash is a very fast game and you must be fit for it – several people have had heart attacks on the squash court because they over-estimated their fitness and ignored chest pains. If you have not played squash before or are coming back to the game after a long absence, you may need some practice on your own to build up your fitness. You will need a lot of carbohydrate – squash uses ten times as much energy as sitting relaxing.

Outward Bound® courses

Since 1984 I have been supervising Outward Bound courses for diabetics over twenty-five. Many participants are over forty – some over sixty years. These courses are run by Outward Bound Eskdale (a member of Outward Bound Trust). Activities include rock climbing, abseiling, canoeing, orienteering, initiative exercises, camping and mountain expeditions. Participants complete a full Outward Bound course without their diabetes getting in the way and without losing control of their blood glucose. At the same time, they learn more about their diabetes, gain in self-confidence and thoroughly enjoy themselves.

Take your pick

There are hundreds of sports to try, whether you are a loner or a team member, whether you want vigorous or gentle exercise. If you choose one which is unfamiliar and potentially hazardous make sure you have a trained instructor (national organisations will guide you) and that you cannot become hypoglycaemic at a critical moment. Make full use of blood-glucose testing to check how you are getting on (see Chapter 8).

Exercise for the elderly

There is no reason why someone over seventy should not enjoy some of the kinds of exercise already described. However, some older people have stiff arthritic joints and a few may be unable to move around easily or be confined to bed. This does not stop you from exercising, though.

The first step is to keep all your joints and ligaments supple. Start at the top of your body and work down. Stretch the muscles of your face by pulling faces; gently turn your neck from side to side and look up and down (do not do this if you have an arthritic neck); flex and straighten your back; pull your abdominal muscles in and out; gently take your arms and legs through the fullest range of movement comfortably possible. Do the breathing exercises described below.

Then, depending on your degree of mobility, try some repetitive exercises – raising and lowering your arms; flexing and extending your legs while sitting; making bicycling movements; or just walking around the room or garden. *The Diabetics' Get Fit Book* by Jackie Winter and Dr Barbara Boucher – gives exercises suitable for older people.

Relaxation

We live in a stress-filled world. Everyone is under some sort of pressure. To survive comfortably we must learn to cope with stress. If we do not we just get more and more wound up and our bodies gradually start to show the strain – ulcers, heart disease, irritable bowel disease, migraine can all be produced or worsened by stress. Diabetes is no exception. Developing the condition in the first place is a stressful event. It seems unlikely that the disease can actually be caused by stress or a shock, although this can raise the blood glucose in someone with a diabetic tendency. People with diabetes may all find that stress upsets their blood glucose control, usually raising the glucose, although something that causes a marked physical reaction may induce a hypoglycaemic attack. Stress causes the release of adrenaline (epinephrine) and noradrenaline (norepinephrine), both of which cause glucose release from the liver.

Elizabeth is forty-three years old and has looked after her diabetes carefully for eight years, with a diabetic diet and one glibenclamide pill daily. Her daughter developed a psychiatric illness. The psychiatric condition worsened and her daughter began to behave bizarrely at home. Elizabeth was naturally very worried and frightened by this and her blood glucose remained over 10 mmol/l – most unusual for her. During the family crisis Elizabeth increased her glibenclamide to one pill twice, then three times, a day after discussions with her doctor. Her daughter recovered with psychiatric treatment and Elizabeth has been able to reduce her glibenclamide dose again.

Breathing exercises

Most of us forget our lungs until they let us down and leave us gasping. Every day, preferably as part of an exercise and relaxation programme, take five minutes to do breathing exercises to open up every part of your lungs and clear any phlegm.

Stand upright, shoulders back in a well-ventilated room. Take in a slow, deep breath filling the whole of your lungs from bottom to top. Pause for a moment then breathe out slowly and carefully, expelling the air from every corner of your lungs. Repeat these deep breaths, practising your control over your diaphragm and chest muscles until you have mastered even inspiration and expiration. Do this slowly – you will get dizzy if you overbreathe. Explore your breathing control. As you breathe out feel all the tension drain from your body.

Use these breathing exercises to unwind when you get angry or upset. Instead of composing abuse about the ancestry and probable fate of the man whose appalling driving has just caused you to brake suddenly, take some deep breaths and let the tension escape.

Another book from Vermilion can help you learn to relax – *Stress and Relaxation* by Jane Madders.

Summary

- Exercise is good for people with diabetes.
- You need the right balance of glucose and insulin to exercise.
- Regular exercise will help you to lose weight and become more sensitive to insulin.
- Check with the doctor that it is safe to exercise.
- Get fit carefully and gradually. Listen to your body and do not hurt yourself.
- Choose exercise you enjoy and do it regularly.
- Learn how to relax and reduce stress.

6

Oral hypoglycaemic pills

Many people with maturity-onset type diabetes will be able to keep their blood glucose under control by diet alone. If this does not return the blood glucose to normal the next step is pill treatment. These pills are called oral (taken by mouth) hypoglycaemic agents (hypo = low and glycaemia = blood glucose).

This chapter describes oral hypoglycaemic pills in some detail – most of the over-forties who need treatment in addition to a diabetic diet and exercise will be taking them. If you are taking medication it is important that you know what it is for, how it works, how much to take and when, and what unwanted effects it may have. It is important to bear in mind that the majority of people do *not* experience side effects of drugs, so do not imagine symptoms!

Your oral hypoglycaemic treatment will be prescribed by your doctor and it is important that you liaise closely with him. I have suggested that it is possible for you to adjust your hypoglycaemic treatment yourself, but this should only be done after prior discussion with your doctor. There may be factors in your particular case which make it inadvisable to vary your treatment. In general the best dose to take is the smallest one that works, i.e. controls the blood glucose. You should not exceed the maximum recommended dose. Practice varies in different countries and drug preparations and the way they are taken may be different; names vary widely. Each drug has a chemical name which is the one you should learn, and a drug company name; for example, glipizide is a chemical name, while Minodiab and Glibenese are the names given to glipizide by two different companies which manufacture it. I have used chemical names throughout this book to avoid confusion.

Sulphonylureas

In the 1950s it was discovered that sulphonylurea drugs lowered the blood glucose. This was a great step forward because until then everyone who could not control their diabetes by diet had to take insulin injections. The first sulphonylurea drug to be marketed extensively as a hypoglycaemic treatment was chlorpropamide. Others are glibenclamide, glipizide, gliquidone, glibornuride, glymidine, tolbutamide, tolazamide and acetohexamide.

Acetohexamide

USA only. Taken before meals – either all at once before breakfast or in divided doses. Maximum daily dose 1500 mg. Medium acting.

Chlorpropamide

Taken once daily with breakfast. Maximum daily dose 500 mg. Very long acting.

Glibenclamide or glyburide

Usually taken in divided doses before meals although the manufacturer suggests once daily with or immediately after breakfast or the first main meal. Maximum daily dose 15 mg. Long acting.

Glibornuride

Taken with breakfast if a small dose; in divided doses with 50 mg with breakfast and the rest with the evening meal if a larger dose. Maximum daily dose 75 mg. Medium acting.

Gliclazide

Taken in two divided doses with the main meals of the day. Maximum daily dose 320 mg. Medium acting.

Glipizide

Taken about 30 minutes before meals. Doses over 15 mg divided between breakfast and lunch and/or evening meal. Maximum daily dose 40 mg. Medium acting.

Gliquidone

Taken up to half an hour before a meal in two or three divided doses, of which the largest dose is usually taken with breakfast. Maximum daily dose 180 mg. Short acting.

Tolbutamide

Taken with or just before meals in single or divided doses. Maximum daily dose 2000 mg. Short acting.

Tolazamide

Taken in divided doses with meals. Maximum daily dose 1000 mg. Medium acting.

At present authorities vary as to the best time to take some glucose-lowering pills. Ask your doctor about your pills.

When not to use sulphonylurea drugs

Sulphonylurea drugs are not recommended in pregnancy because it is not known whether they will cause malformations in the baby. They should not be taken by breast-feeding mothers. Because they are broken down by the liver they should be used with caution or not at all in people with liver damage. The breakdown products and any remaining active drug are passed out in the urine, so care is also required in people with kidney damage. In both liver and kidney damage a small dose of sulphonylurea may cause unexpected hypoglycaemia. The drugs should also be used with caution in people with adrenal insufficiency and thyroid disease.

Drug interactions

Hypoglycaemia may occur because of interference in the way in which some sulphonylurea drugs are carried in the blood or broken down. Interacting drugs include sulphonamide antibiotics, phenylbutazone, aspirin, probenecid, coumarin anti-coagulants (warfarin), beta blockers, chloramphenicol, monoamine oxidase inhibitors and sulphinpyrazone. Some drugs such as thiazide diuretics or steroids may increase the blood glucose. Sulphonylureas may prolong the effect of barbiturates.

Side effects

These are uncommon. Sulphonylureas may, like any drug, cause allergic reactions producing a variety of skin rashes. These usually settle when the drug is stopped. Sulphonylureas may also cause gastrointestinal symptoms such as loss of appetite, nausea, vomiting, indigestion and diarrhoea or constipation. These are usually mild and dose dependent and settle if the dose is reduced or divided. Potentially more serious but rare side effects are liver damage, occasionally causing jaundice; and abnormalities of the blood cells. These usually improve when the drug is stopped.

A drink of alcohol causes flushing in about 60 per cent of all patients taking chlorpropamide and and may do so in those on other sulphonylurea drugs. This effect is sometimes unpleasant but nearly always harmless (6 per cent of the population flush with alcohol anyway). Chlorpropamide has another unusual action which is not shared by other sulphonylurea drugs. It acts like anti-diuretic hormone to conserve water in the body and can actually be used to treat diabetes insipidus (see page 11). Chlorpropamide may lower the blood sodium level, especially in people on diuretic tablets.

A further factor which should be mentioned is the

University Group Diabetes program (UGDP) study performed in the USA in the 1960s. This study was cut short
because early analysis seemed to show a higher death rate
from heart disease in a group of patients treated with
tolbutamide than in those on other treatment. This led to a
move away from sulphonylureas in America, but subse-
quently some of the design and conclusions of the UGDP
study were criticised. Other studies did not support the
UGDP findings. Most British doctors and many American
doctors continue to prescribe sulphonylureas because there
is no clear evidence to indicate that they are harmful in the
majority of people. The UK Prospective Diabetes Study may
provide some clarification when it finishes.

How do sulphonylureas work?

Sulphonylurea drugs produce a hypoglycaemic effect only in
people who can still make some of their own insulin. They
increase the amount of insulin released from the pancreas as
the blood glucose rises after a meal. In addition they reduce
the resistance to insulin action at cell level, possibly by
increasing insulin binding at tissue receptors.

Which sulphonylurea?

There is a bewildering number of sulphonylurea drugs.
How does your doctor choose which one to give you? The
honest answer is the one he/she is most familiar with – and
this may well be one of the older ones like glibenclamide. But
there are other factors to consider, an important one being the
duration of action of the drug. Chlorpropamide is the
longest-acting sulphonylurea – which means that it is useful
in providing all-round action after one dose a day. However,
if too much is given or too little food is eaten, the person may
be hypoglycaemic for a very long time. Thus it can be useful
in younger pill-treated diabetics but is not advisable in
elderly people or those with any kidney damage. Short-
acting sulphonylureas may give more flexibility in meal
times and quantities.

Biguanides

Metformin is the only biguanide oral hypoglycaemic drug in current use in most countries. The maximum daily dose is 3000 mg daily, although most British physicians would not increase the dose above 1500 mg in twenty-four hours. It is taken before or with meals in divided doses.

When not to use metformin

Metformin is contraindicated in pregnancy and lactation, and it should be used with care in people over sixty-five years old. Metformin should not be given to people with kidney or liver damage, nor to people who have had a recent heart attack or who drink excessive alcohol at any time. It should also be avoided in people with severe chest or heart trouble who have a low blood-oxygen level.

Drug interactions

Like the sulphonylureas, metformin may interact with coumarin anticoagulants (warfarin), in this case upsetting the blood-clotting control.

Side effects

Metformin commonly causes gastrointestinal symptoms when treatment is first started – particularly loss of appetite, nausea and diarrhoea. These usually settle as the body gets used to the drug, but if not the dose can be temporarily reduced. The most serious side effect of biguanides, however, is lactic acidosis. This led to metformin's predecessor, phenformin, being withdrawn in many countries. Metformin is much safer than phenformin. Lactic acidosis is a condition in which waste acids build up in the blood, and can be fatal. It is rare with metformin and occurs mainly in patients with the contraindications above. It is the reason why people taking metformin should avoid alcohol if possible, and should certainly never get drunk.

How does metformin work in diabetes?

In people with diabetes, metformin lowers the blood glucose towards normal but rarely causes hypoglycaemia on its own. In non-diabetics the blood glucose level is unchanged. Metformin probably reduces glucose absorption from the gut and increases glucose uptake by the tissues. It also improves insulin binding to receptors.

When to use metformin

Metformin is advocated for people with diabetes who are overweight and who have been unable to control their blood glucose by diet alone. Some physicians think that such patients lose more weight on diet and metformin treatment than on sulphonylurea and diet treatment.

Metformin may be added to the treatment of people whose blood glucose has failed to return to normal on sulphony-lurea and diet. This double oral hypoglycaemic treatment is sometimes successful in controlling the blood glucose.

Problems with pill taking

To be effective the right dose of pills should be taken every day at the times your doctor recommends. Use a calendar box (see page 143), or set out each day's pills in the morning, or use a checklist. If you are on once-daily pills and miss your morning dose, take it later if you remember within four hours. If you forget until next day just take your normal dose then – do *not* take double to try and make up! You should *never* exceed the maximum daily dose. So, take the right number of pills – not too few and not too many – at the right time.

Most pills are marketed by several different companies and in different strengths. It is therefore important to know the *dose* you are taking. For example, it is not much use telling a new doctor you are taking one chlorpropamide a day; this could mean a daily dose of 100 mg or 250 mg, as the drug is marketed in both strengths.

If you think that your pills are upsetting you in any way, stop them and contact your family doctor or the person who prescribed them straightaway. Do not just stop them and do nothing. Do not carry on if you fear that they are not suiting you. Discuss it with an expert!

Hypoglycaemia or a low blood glucose

Hypoglycaemia may occur with sulphonylureas, but is rare with metformin. It is probably commoner than people realise, although rarely a severe problem. Sulphonylurea treatment should always be started cautiously, especially in older people as they are sometimes very sensitive to small doses. Glibenclamide may be especially likely to cause hypoglycaemia in the elderly.

The symptoms of a low blood glucose include tiredness, feeling muddled, sweaty, tingly, hungry, dizzy or light-headed, palpitations, altered perception, clumsiness, irritation, euphoria, slurred speech. If you feel like this or unusual in any other way, especially after your first dose of sulphonylurea, before a meal or after exercise check your blood glucose (see page 68). If it is low, i.e. below 4 mmol/l (72 mg/dl) eat something sweet straightaway. Glucose is fastest, but a sugary drink, sweet or candy, biscuit or piece of bread will get your glucose level up too.

If you cannot check your blood or are in doubt about the result of the test, eat something anyway. Then have a proper meal with plenty of high-fibre carbohydrate. This is important because the sulphonylurea drug will have 'primed' your pancreas to release insulin so that when you eat the glucose too much insulin may be released, making you hypoglycaemic again. When you feel better contact your diabetes adviser. Do not take any more of your sulphonylurea pills until you have spoken with him.

Sick days

Pills that you take by mouth rely on a normal gastrointestinal tract to reach the bloodstream. If they are not absorbed they cannot work. Illnesses that make you vomit or have diarrhoea may mean that you do not absorb your pills. When you are ill your body releases hormones to help you to recover. These hormones tend to increase the blood glucose. This means that someone on pills who develops gastroenteritis may find that their blood glucose is rising fast.

If you have vomited within two hours of taking your hypoglycaemic pills, take the same dose again. If these do not stay down and your blood glucose is rising (see Chapter 8 on glucose measuring) call your doctor straightaway. You may need to have insulin injections temporarily until you recover. When you are ill drink plenty of fluids – small amounts frequently is often best.

Acarbose

Dose 50 mg three times a day. After six to eight weeks this dose can be increased gradually to 100 mg three times a day. The maximum dose is 200 mg three times a day.

When we eat sugary or starchy foods, their carbohydrates are broken down into simple carbohydrates like glucose. Acarbose blocks this effect, thereby reducing the amount of glucose available for absorption into the bloodstream.

Acarbose has yet to be widely used in Britain but is used elsewhere in Europe. It can improve blood glucose balance in people whose diabetes is not controlled on diet alone, or may be added to sulphonylurea treatment. If you are taking both acarbose and a sulphonylurea pill you must carry glucose (dextrose) to treat hypoglycaemia. Sucrose (ordinary sugar) will not work as your body will not be able to digest it into glucose.

The main side effect of acarbose is an excess of bowel gas produced as unabsorbed carbohydrate ferments. This can be uncomfortable and embarrassing and will be worse if you are eating a lot of sugar.

Summary

- Sulphonylurea or biguanide oral hypoglycaemic pills are a useful adjunct to diet and exercise treatment in diabetes.
- There are many different sulphonylurea drugs – learn all about the one you are taking.

- Avoid excess alcohol.
- Take your pills as instructed. Consult your doctor if you are unhappy about any aspect of your drug treatment.
- Watch your blood glucose especially carefully if you are ill. Contact your diabetes adviser if your glucose is high or you think you are not absorbing your pills.
- Remember that hypoglycaemia can occur with pills.
- Check the recommendations in this chapter with your doctor.

7

Insulin

Insulin is a protein. It cannot be given by mouth as it is attacked and broken down by the digestive enzymes in the gut. Research work is going on to find ways of protecting insulin from these enzymes by coating it in other, enzyme-resistant, substances. Insulin nasal sprays have also been developed. However, neither of these methods is generally available and both have a lot of problems which need to be overcome. The generally available method of administration of insulin is therefore by injection.

Some of you will have been taking insulin since childhood or early teens. This means that you have insulin deficiency; your pancreas stopped making insulin many years ago. Some of you, however, will have come to insulin treatment after diet and oral hypoglycaemic drugs have failed to control the blood glucose. You may have started off with an insulin-resistance problem and gradually become insulin deficient. And some of my readers will have gone to their doctor with insulin-deficient diabetes over the age of thirty.

The different ways in which people come to insulin treatment influence their attitudes to it. If you have never had an alternative to insulin it is sometimes easier to accept it than if you have had a period of pill treatment first. On the other hand, failure to control your blood glucose on diet and pills makes you unwell (whether you realise it or not) and insulin treatment will give you an enormous improvement in physical well-being. It is never worth struggling on with high blood-glucose levels on pills merely because you are nervous about going on to insulin injections – they are no more painful than a gnat bite and if children of four can give themselves their own insulin so can you.

Whichever situation you find yourself in, the important thing to accept is that your blood glucose can now be controlled only by insulin injections.

Types of insulin

Human insulin has a unique chemical structure. It is what all human beings make unless they develop diabetes. However, for over fifty years of insulin therapy people with diabetes had to make do with insulin derived from pig or beef pancreas. It then became possible to manufacture human insulin by genetic modification of bacteria or yeasts, and by chemical modification of pork insulin.

Nowadays, most people use human insulin. There are still some people injecting pork insulin and a few on beef insulin. The latter often require large doses of insulin to overcome the antibodies that their body's immune system makes to fight the 'foreign insulin'. Pork insulin can also cause antibody formation, although usually to a lesser degree. Some people who change from animal to human insulin feel that they have less warning of hypoglycaemia after the change. Careful scientific studies have shown no significant difference in the symptoms or signs of hypoglycaemia when such people have been given human or animal insulins without knowing which is which. However, you must feel that you are on the treatment that suits you best – after all, you are the one who has to inject it. If you are still using animal insulin you will have had diabetes for many years and you will be familiar with your insulin and how it works for you. There is rarely any need to change to human insulin unless you want to. Remember, though, that the passage of time may alter the way in which you respond to your insulin, including reducing your warning of hypoglycaemia.

Rapid acting

Pure insulin is a clear colourless fluid. This is what your body was making before you became diabetic. If injected into a vein it starts to reduce the blood glucose within minutes. If injected under the skin (subcutaneously) it starts to act within half an hour and lasts eight hours at most. This clear form of insulin is called soluble or regular insulin, and is the fast-acting form. Some examples are Actrapid, Velosulin, Humulin S (R USA).

Most people need rapid-acting insulin at breakfast time and some like to take it before each meal. It copes with the glucose absorbed from the meal.

Longer acting

Longer-acting insulins contain protamine and/or zinc to slow down absorption and duration of action. Amorphous (semilente) or crystalline (ultralente) insulins are also available. Because of the addition of other chemicals or the alteration in structure all longer-acting insulins are cloudy. Some medium-to longer-acting insulins are Semitard, NPH (neutral protamine Hagedorn), Humulin I, Insulatard, Monotard, Lentard, Humulin Zn. The longest-acting insulins are Ultratard, Protamine Zinc Insulin and Hypurin Lente.

Very long-acting insulins provide background action for glucose 'housekeeping' between meals. Medium-acting insulin taken before breakfast may also reduce the lunchtime glucose peak. Some people take fast-acting insulin before each meal and medium- (or long) active insulin prebed.

Mixtures

If you wish you can inject fast and slow insulins separately as often as necessary each day. However, it is more comfortable to mix these insulins in the syringe and give them as one injection at each time of day. Twice daily is usually sufficient. However, remember that mixtures of medium and fast insulin are relatively stable but that mixtures of slower and fast insulin may not be. Preferably all home-mixed injections should be given within fifteen minutes of mixing.

Some fixed-proportion mixtures are available from manufacturers. These include Mixtard (30:70 fast:medium and Initard 50:50), Humulin M1 (10:90), Humulin M2

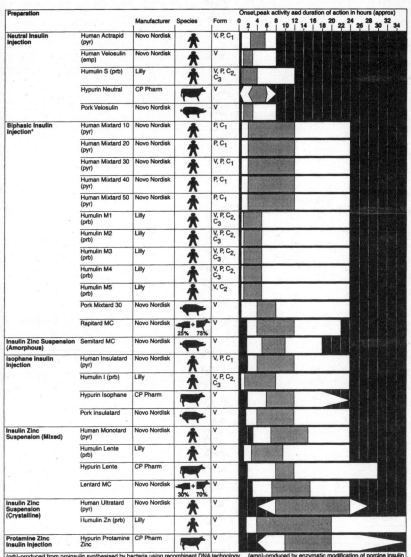

Duration of action of different insulins. (Reproduced by courtesy of MIMS magazine, May 1996.)

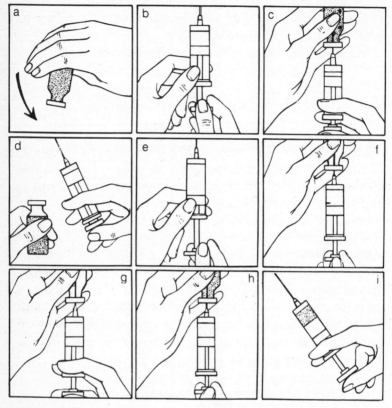

a) Gently rotate bottle to mix insulin
b) Draw up air
c) Inject air into cloudy insulin bottle
d) Put cloudy insulin down
e) Draw up air

f) Inject air into clear insulin bottle. Draw up clear insulin
g) Express air bubbles and check you have drawn up correct dose of clear insulin
h) Draw up correct dose of cloudy insulin
i) Ready for injection

Mixing fast- and slow-acting insulins in the syringe.

(20:80), Humulin M3 (30:70), Humulin M4 (40:60) Humulin M5 (50:50). Humulin insulins are available in cartridges for pens. The Penmix range is available as cartridges or in preloaded disposable insulin pens (Penmix 10:90, 20:80, 30:70, 40:60 and 50:50). If you have a similar food and exercise routine each day you may find such a ready-made mixture helpful. I also find them useful in people who cannot see very well and in those who are still making a little of their own insulin. Fixed-proportion mixtures may suit elderly people.

However they may not suit people with a very varied lifestyle, because they are inflexible.

Make sure you know which insulin you take.

Practicalities of insulin administration

The insulin bottle

Most insulin comes in bottles with a self-sealing rubber bung. Clean the bung before drawing up, if it has got dirty. Some insulins also come in cartridges for use in insulin pens and or in preloaded pens Velosulin comes in vials for use in insulin pumps. All insulin should be stored in the fridge at 2–8°C and never heated or frozen. It will not go off if carried at body temperature when used in pumps or pens.

Always check the type of insulin and expiry date before drawing up. All insulin in the UK and USA is marketed at a strength of 100 units per ml (U100). Some other countries still use 40 units per ml (U40) or 80 units per ml (U80). Beware confusion if you have to get insulin abroad – better still take what you need with you.

Syringes and needles

The simplest way to give insulin is using a syringe and needle. The best syringes and needles are the disposable ones; they are accurate and virtually painless. Most people with diabetes reuse their disposable syringes and needles for several days. This practice is not thought to be associated with any greater risk of infection than from glass syringes; however, the manufacturers do recommend single use only. Glass syringes are hard to keep clean (use industrial methylated spirits and boil intermittently), may become inaccurate and break.

Click-count syringes, with an audible click for every two units of insulin, are available for people with poor vision, as are magnifiers for ordinary syringes (e.g. C-Better, Char-Mag, Magni-Guide, Syringe Magnifier). Preset syringes can also be used (e.g. Andros IDM, B-D Cornwall, Dos-Aid,

Insulgage). None of these devices remove the problem of a
person with poor vision drawing up air rather than insulin.
Drawing-up aids include 'Centre Point' Funnel, Holdease,
Inject-Aid, Injection Safety Guard, Insulin Aid and Insulin
Needle Guide and Location Tray.

Injection technique

If you are well padded, with plenty of fatty tissue under the
skin (subcutaneously), all you need to do is push the needle
in at right angles to the skin and inject. Slimmer people may

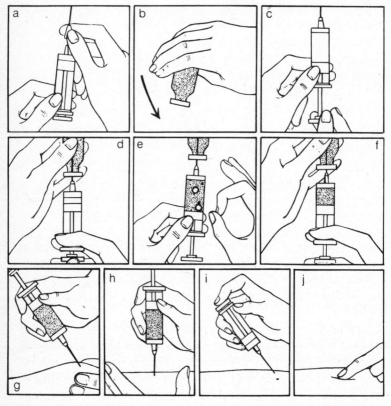

a) Attach needle to syringe if necessary
b) Gently rotate bottle to mix insulin
c) Draw up air and inject into the insulin bottle
d) Draw up insulin
e) Clear air bubbles

f) Check syringe contains correct insulin
   dose
g+h) Inject insulin into fatty layer under skin
i) Withdraw needle
j) Press on the hole

Drawing up insulin and injecting it.

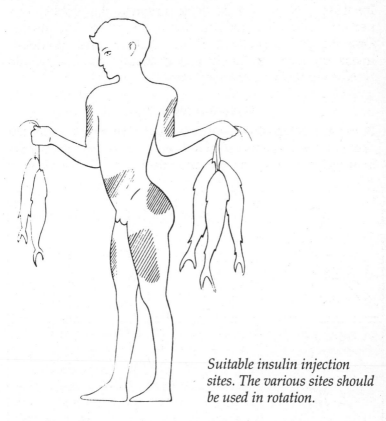

Suitable insulin injection sites. The various sites should be used in rotation.

need to pinch up some skin and very slim people may need to slant the needle to ensure that the insulin enters subcutaneous fat and not muscle. Do not swab with alcohol unless your skin is dirty and you cannot use soap and water and a clean towel.

Injecting in and out fast is most comfortable. Use the various injection sites around the body in turn, in order to avoid lumps and dents which can occur if you use the same area repeatedly (see page 134). And remember that muscle activity under the injection site, or another form of warming, may increase the insulin absorption rate (e.g. running after injecting in the thigh). Injection aids include Auto Injector, Hypoguard Automatic Injector, Instaject and Palmer injection gun. They are rarely needed.

Timing and patterns of insulin administration

Give most insulins 20–30 minutes before meals. The two common patterns of insulin therapy are:

- fast- and medium-acting twice a day (morning fast-acting for breakfast until lunchtime, morning medium-acting for lunch until evening meal; evening fast-acting for evening meal until bed, evening medium-acting for overnight until next morning);
- long-acting once or twice a day or very long-acting insulin once a day to act as background, with fast-acting insulin before breakfast, possibly before lunch and before evening meal.

What is best for you?

You need to discuss your lifestyle, food and exercise pattern with your diabetes adviser. Often people who have changed from pill treatment to insulin can manage with less day-to-day variation in insulin dose and are well controlled on fixed-proportion mixtures. They are usually buffering the insulin action by being overweight, as well as making a little of their own insulin. People who are totally insulin deficient tend to need flexible insulin regimens which they can adjust for activities at any time of day. They may find that the dose and timing are critical. It is always possible to find the insulin regimen that suits you even if it takes some trial and error for the first few months.

Other ways of giving insulin

Insulin pens

Nowadays there are several pen injection devices available. More and more people are using them because they are portable, easy to use and accurate, and injections are often more comfortable than with a conventional needle and syringe. However, the pens are heavier and thicker than syringes and some people find them harder to manage. In insulin pens the ink cartridge is replaced with an insulin cartridge and the nib with a disposable double-ended needle, one end to inject the insulin subcutaneously, the other end to pierce the insulin cartridge. Pens have a scale to dial up the dose of insulin you need. Some pens only allow increments of two units, others one unit. Some pens will allow bigger maximum doses of insulin than others. Most pens have a window to see how much insulin you have left.

Each pen can be used only with the insulin produced by that pen manufacturer. Pens use human insulin – there are no pens for pork or beef insulin. Pens include the BD range (takes Humulin range of cartridges, e.g. Humulin S, Humulin M1 to M5) and the NovoNordisk range (takes Penfill cartridges such as Actrapid, Insulatard and the Penmix range). Novo Nordisk also produce disposable, preloaded insulin pens containing Actrapid, Insulatard and Penmix 10:90 to 50:50 insulins). Diapen is an automatic pen-injection costing £50.

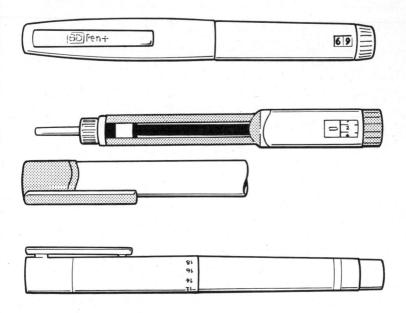

Three types of insulin pen syringes.

Insulin jets

These large machines drive a high-pressure jet of insulin
through the skin without requiring a needle. It sounds a good
idea but they are not always accurate and are cumbersome to
use. However, if someone has needle phobia this may solve
the problem. The machines, e.g. Preci-jet 50, are rarely used
in Britain; Medijector and Vitajet are American models.

Insulin pumps

Continuous subcutaneous insulin infusion (CSII) is one way
of mimicking normal insulin release by the pancreas. Rapid-
acting insulin in a vial or syringe is pumped continuously
through a tube to a needle left under the skin for one or two
days. At meal times extra insulin boosts are given. Modern
pumps are small (about the size of two matchboxes) and light
and many have very sophisticated controls. However, unlike
the real pancreas they cannot tell what the blood glucose
level is. The wearer has to do that by a finger-prick test at least
four times a day. Needle glucose-sensors are being developed to feed signals straight back to the pumps, but at the
moment they are still at the research stage.

CSII is not a simple answer. It needs constant vigilance and
provides no better control than carefully-monitored frequent
injections. The pump is always attached to you and some
people find the needle under the skin uncomfortable. However, others find that the increased flexibility of continuous
insulin, with meal-time boosts as needed, makes their lives
easier.

If you do decide to try a pump, discuss it thoroughly with
your adviser first. Then borrow one to try before buying
(they are expensive). If you use CSII you must have twenty-
four-hour access to a pump expert in case of problems. I have
not named examples of such pumps as I believe it is vitally
important that any CSII pump is obtained only through a
doctor.

Summary

- If you are over forty you may always have needed insulin therapy or you may come to need it after a trial of pill treatment.
- Once it has become obvious that you need insulin, accept it and learn to handle it.
- There are many different insulin treatments. Ask your diabetes adviser to help you to choose the one that suits you and your lifestyle.
- Learn everything you can about your insulins and how they work in you.
- Learn precisely how best to inject your insulin. Consider different ways of administering insulin if you have difficulties. Find out about modern advances in injection therapy, but only change if the new method offers distinct advantages.

8

Blood-glucose control

Everyone with diabetes should aim to keep his or her blood glucose within the normal range, that is between 4 and 7.8 mmol/l (72 to 140 mg/dl). However, no one with diabetes will succeed in doing this all the time; you have to balance the effort of trying to do this against the short- and long-term benefits. In the short term you will feel better with a normal glucose level; in the long term, as I discuss later, keeping your blood glucose normal reduces the risk of diabetic tissue damage. If you find that frequent finger-prick glucose measurements or frequent hypoglycaemic attacks due to overtight glucose control interfere with your enjoyment of life you may feel that some compromise is appropriate. However, it is important to do your best to keep your blood glucose normal for as much of the time as possible.

Blood-glucose measurement

Why measure the blood glucose? In Chapter 3 I described how to check the urine for glucose. This will give you an approximate idea of what is happening to your blood glucose over the time that the urine was filtering through the kidneys and being collected in the bladder. But everyone has a slightly different kidney threshold for glucose – some people filter more glucose into the urine than others, and your kidney threshold may change over the years. Nowadays, most diabetics know how to measure urine glucose but rely mainly on direct blood-glucose measurement for monitoring.

The principle behind blood-glucose testing is that the

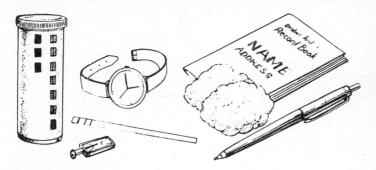

Blood-glucose testing. You will need . ...

glucose in a tiny drop of blood from a finger-prick reacts with chemicals in a pad on the end of a strip. As it reacts the chemicals change colour; usually, the darker the colour the more glucose in the blood. Different manufacturers use different colour ranges – thus BM strips (Chemstrips bG USA) are blue and beige-green, Dextrostix are grey-purple, Glucostix are yellow-green and orange. Other makes are Hypoguard and Hypoguard GA. Choose the colours which you find easiest to see. Exactech is a biosensor which does not require colour matching, wiping or blotting. Place the strip in the sensor, drop the blood on the strip, press the start button, and the result is displayed digitally in thirty seconds. (MediSens card turns itself on and takes 20 seconds.) You cannot check the result by looking at the strip, so accurate technique is essential, and you must follow the manufacturer's instructions exactly as with all blood-testing systems. Once you have done the test write the result down in a diabetic diary.

Finger pricking

There are many devices on the market to make finger-pricking (finger-sticking for American readers) easier. See table of lancets and finger prickers, overleaf. However, you do not have to have a special device – a simple lancet will do (e.g. Ames Lancet, B-D Microfine, Monolet or Unilet).

It is easier to obtain a good drop of blood if your hands are warm. Prick the fingers you use least, or, as some people do,

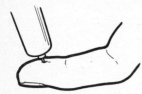

Prick clean warm finger to obtain a big drop of blood. A finger - pricking device is better than a lancet alone.

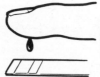

Drop blood on to stick covering test pad completely. Do not rub or smudge.

 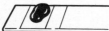

Leave drop on test pad for specified time (check manufacturer's instructions)

Clean blood from test pad and wait extra time (check manufacturer's instructions)

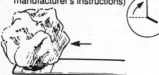

Wipe, e.g. BM-test - 1 - 44

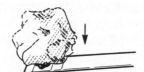

Blot e.g. Glucostix.

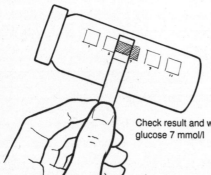

Check result and write it down, e.g. 4pm blood glucose 7 mmol/l

Measuring blood glucose.

Finger Prickers and Compatible Lancets

Compatible Lancets	Finger Pricking Devices*									
	Autoclix	Auto Lancet	Autolet	Autolet Lite	B-D Lancer	Glucolet	Hypolet	Monojector	Penlet II	Soft Touch
Ames			•	•	•					
B-D Microfine +		•			•	•		•	•	•
Cleanlet 25	•	•	•	•	•	•	•	•	•	•
Cleanlet 25XL			•	•	•					
Monolet	•	•	•	•	•	•	•	•	•	•
Monolet Extra			•	•	•					
Unilet Superlite			•	•	•					
Unilet Superlite G	•	•						•	•	•
Unilet Universal			•	•	•	•	•	•	•	•

*N.B.: Finger pricking devices are not prescribable at NHS expense.

Reproduced courtesy of MIMS, May 1996.

use the ear lobe. You should ensure that your anti-tetanus vaccinations are up to date, especially if you have an outdoor job or work with animals, and you should wash your hands well in warm water before you test.

BLOOD GLUCOSE TESTING STRIPS AND METERS

Meter	Sensitivity Range (mmol/l)	Manufacturer	Retail Price (exc. VAT)	BM Accutest	BM Test 1-44	ExacTech	G2	Glucostix	Glucotide	Hypoguard GA	Hypoguard Supreme	One Touch	Medi-Test Glycaemic C
Accutrend	1·1-33·3	B.M. Diag	£34·00	•									
Accutrend Alpha	1·1-27·8	B.M. Diag	£29·00	•									
Accutrend DM	1·1-33·33	B.M. Diag	£149·00	•									
Accutrend GC*	1·1-33·3	B.M. Diag	£199·00	•									
Accutrend Mini	1·67-22·2	B.M. Diag	£25·00	•									
Exac Tech	2·2-25	Medi Sense	£24·00			•							
Glucometer 4	0·6-33·3	Bayer	£35·00					•					
Glycotronic C	1·1-33·3	BHR	£31·00										•
Hypocount Supreme	2-22·0	Hypoguard (UK)	£34·95								•		
Hypocount GA	0-22·0	Hypoguard (UK)	£24·95							•			
One Touch Basic	0-33·3	Lifescan	£39·00									•	
One Touch II	0-33·3	Lifescan	£59·00									•	
MediSense Card	1·1-33·3	Medi Sense	£35·00				•						
MediSense Pen	1·1-33·3	Medi Sense	£35·00				•						
Reflolux S	0·5-27·7	B.M. Diag.	£29·00		•								

● Meters are not available at NHS expense.   *Combined Glucose/Cholesterol Meter

Reproduced courtesy of MIMS, May 1996.

Meters

Used carefully, precisely according to instructions, visually-read blood-testing strips are virtually as accurate as a meter. However, colour-blind people and those with diabetic eye problems have problems matching colours.

Nowadays, many people with diabetes use meters to measure their blood glucose level. Some meters take the strips used for visual reading, others have strips solely for meter use. Follow the instructions very carefully. Wrong procedure = wrong result. When choosing a meter, look at several before purchase. Your meter should be easy for you to use – think about the number of steps you have to remember, how easy it might be to make a mistake, the speed and readability of the result. Is the device portable, robust, easy to clean? Does it have a memory or not?

Remember that it is no use having elaborate technology to measure your blood glucose concentration if you do not take action on the results. Make sure you learn how to adjust your treatment so that you can safely improve your blood glucose concentrations. In other words, 'Don't just sit there, do something!'

Hypoglycaemia

What is hypoglycaemia?

If your blood glucose level is below 4 mmol/l (72 mg/dl) you are hypoglycaemic.

Your brain needs glucose to function. As the glucose level falls you may start to feel muddled, develop altered perception, become uncoordinated, slur your speech, get irritable, become tearful or laugh, feel tingling and, if you are hypoglycaemic for a long time, eventually become drowsy and lose consciousness. Long before this happens your body will arouse its defence mechanisms. Adrenaline (epinephrine) and steroid hormones pour out of the adrenal glands to help raise the blood glucose. The adrenaline (epinephrine) makes you sweat and feel frightened (it is the fright, flight and fight hormone). Your heart races and your skin may change colour. Other names for this state are 'hypo', insulin reaction, a 'low', a 'turn' – and one of my patients calls her hypoglycaemic episodes 'whoopsies'! I know what she means but other people do not, and it is better to use the proper name so that everyone knows what you are talking about. People with solely diet-treated diabetes do not develop hypoglycaemia.

The cure – glucose

The instant cure for all these symptoms is glucose. In an emergency anything sweet and sugary will work, but glucose works fastest and is available in many forms; these include glucose gel (Glutose, Hypostop, Monogel), glucose tablets (BD Glucose tablets, Boots' glucose tablets, Dextrosol, Lucozade tablets), glucose powder dissolved in milk, juice or water, and Coca Cola, Pepsi Cola or Lucozade. (NB 'Diet' drinks will not work.) You should always carry glucose and eat some at the first signs of hypoglycaemia. Sometimes people with hypoglycaemia refuse food or glucose because they are confused. The only thing for their friends and family to do is be firm and insist that they eat.

Occasionally, people with diabetes are not aware that they are becoming hypoglycaemic. If this applies to you, ask your family and friends to keep a gentle eye on you, and tell them what to look out for. Check whether you are on medication which may reduce the warning – propranolol and the other beta blocker drugs can do this. If you are, discuss it with your doctor.

Severe hypoglycaemia

Rarely, hypoglycaemia is bad enough to make someone unconscious. This is usually because it has been untreated for many hours. It is frightening for those around you but rarely causes serious harm, so no one should panic.

The first thing to do is put the unconscious person in the recovery position, lying on his side with the airway clear. (Very rarely, convulsions may occur; if so remove hard or sharp objects to prevent injury.) Then ask someone to call the doctor or do so yourself. Then start trying to revive the hypoglycaemic person. Oral glucose may still work, but must be used carefully to prevent choking. Never give oral glucose to someone having a fit. Small amounts of glucose gel or powder rubbed inside the cheek closest to the ground will be absorbed from the mouth.

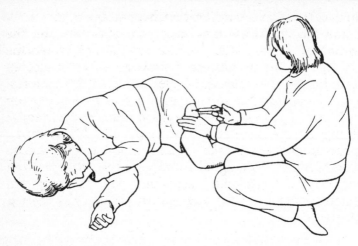

Treating someone unconscious from hypoglycaemia. She is safe lying in the recovery position while you decide what to do. Her companion is about to inject glucagon into the muscles of her thigh. When she has woken up, give her something to eat.

Glucagon

Glucagon is a hormone which raises the blood glucose by releasing liver stores into the circulation. It can be kept at home and relatives can administer it to you if you do become unconscious from hypoglycaemia. It rarely has to be used but it is reassuring to have it in the house.

Glucagon needs to be dissolved in the solvent provided with it, drawn into a syringe and injected deep into a muscle (it also works after intravenous or subcutaneous injection). It is harmless, apart from sometimes causing nausea, vomiting or headache. Glucagon's effect is temporary, so feed the person as soon as they are awake. If you have no glucagon, if it does not work or if fitting occurs call the doctor. Keep the person warm in the recovery position with a clear airway until the doctor comes.

Why were you hypoglycaemic?

If you have a hypoglycaemic attack, make sure that you have had enough to eat and then start to work out why it happened. Did you miss a meal? Have you exercised more than usual? Try to ensure it cannot happen again.

Some factors which may take you unawares are: the lowering of glucose after exercise has finished, when the body reorganises its glucose stores; the effect of alcohol which blocks the release of glucose from liver stores; nocturnal hypoglycaemia if you go to bed with a low glucose (it is better to go to sleep with a blood glucose of 6 mmol/l (108 mg/dl) than one of 4 mmol/l (72 mg/dl); nocturnal hypoglycaemia if you wake up in the morning with glucose levels of 4 mmol/l (72 mg/dl); unexpected exercise due to an emergency. Your insulin needs may fall following the hormonal changes of the menopause, causing unexpected hypoglycaemia.

Hyperglycaemia

Every diabetic will have the occasional 10 or 13 mmol/l reading (180 or 234 mg/dl). This is nothing to worry about, but if your readings are consistently above normal you should do something about it. Are you sticking to your diet? Are you getting enough exercise? Does your insulin or pill dose need increasing? Have you forgotten to take your pills or insulin?

Causes of hyperglycaemia

You may be able to recognise events which will increase your blood glucose, and learn to take preventive action. Obviously eating a larger meal or new foods is a common factor. Menstrual periods in women are often associated with a rise in glucose before, during or after blood loss. (Some women find that they need to change their treatment after the menopause – perhaps reducing their medication.) Getting upset, angry or frightened (i.e. raising your adrenaline) may produce a temporary rise.

Another cause of unexpectedly high glucose levels is infection. Your body again releases defence hormones and the resistance to insulin increases rapidly. This may occur before you actually feel ill.

Ketones

Ketones are produced when someone becomes severely insulin deficient. They are the breakdown products of fat and they make the blood acid. Ketones are also produced during starvation. Ketones are found in insulin-dependent diabetics who are not taking enough insulin for their body's current needs. They are uncommon in people taking oral hypogly-caemic pills but may occur if these are no longer working.

You can test for urinary ketones using test strips (Ketodia-bur, Ketostix, for example). Moderate or large quantities of ketones and blood glucose levels above 13 mmol/l (234 mg/dl) indicate insulin deficiency. If this happens you should contact your doctor. Increase your insulin if you usually have insulin injections.

Sick days – some examples

Rosa Rosa is fifty-two and overweight. She has had diabetes for two years and takes glipizide 5 mg daily. Her job in a baker's shop puts terrible temptations in her way every day. It also means that she stands for much of the time.

Recently her fat cat, Thomas, scratched her leg and an ulcer formed. The ulcer was being cleaned and dressed by the nurse three times a week but one weekend it became infected. Rosa did not realise that this had happened but her blood glucose measurements, which had been under 10 mmol/l (180 mg/dl), started to rise so that they were all above 13 mmol/l (234 mg/dl). Rosa increased her glipizide to 5 mg twice a day on Saturday and three times a day on Sunday and contacted her doctor on Monday. He diagnosed and treated the infection with antibiotics and asked Rosa to stay off work for two weeks. The infection settled rapidly and the ulcer healed once Rosa was off her feet. She kept a close watch on her glucose and gradually reduced the glipizide back to 5 mg daily as the glucose levels returned to normal.

Rosa's prompt action kept her blood glucose levels under control, although in retrospect she should have called the doctor in over the weekend so that the infection could have been treated earlier.

Freda Freda is seventy-two and has been diabetic for ten years, treated with the maximum dose of tolbutamide. She developed ankle swelling due to congestive cardiac failure (see page 95) and her doctor prescribed bendrofluazide (thiazide diuretic) which reduced the swelling.

Next week Freda's grandson came to visit. Unfortunately he had a cold and gave it to Freda, who is prone to chest infections. She started to feel rather poorly and took to her bed. She did not feel like eating or drinking but she took all her pills. She felt too weak to check her urine glucose. Two days after the start of her cold her daughter found her feverish, muddled and very dry and called the doctor. He sent her to hospital where she was found to be extremely dehydrated, with a chest infection and a blood glucose concentration of 54 mmol/l (972 mg/dl). Her urine was loaded with glucose but there were no ketones. She was in a hyperglycaemic dehydrated non-ketotic state (sometimes called a hyperosmolar 'coma'), which is an uncommon but serious condition in which the patient is grossly dehydrated with very high blood glucose levels. In Freda's case this state had been precipitated by the combination of an infection, which raised her blood glucose and made her too unwell to drink properly, and diuretic pills, which raise the blood glucose and cause fluid loss. She recovered with careful fluid replacement and insulin treatment.

In elderly people, several conditions may exist together and a combination of circumstances may add to cause severe illness. Freda should have telephoned her doctor when she started to feel unwell. Everyone with diabetes should have a telephone.

Bob Bob is forty-three years old and has been an insulin-treated diabetic since he was twenty-nine. He works in a factory and is rarely ill.

One night he started to feel shivery, nauseated and ached all over. That morning he began to vomit and had some diarrhoea. Because he was vomiting he was unable to eat and because he was afraid he would become hypoglycaemic he did not give his insulin injection. By evening he was still vomiting and feeling dreadful. He thought he had better omit the evening insulin as well because he had eaten nothing. At 6 am next morning his wife became frightened because he was very drowsy and was breathing oddly. She called the doctor who admitted him to hospital immediately. His urine contained large amounts of glucose and ketones. After insulin and 7 litres of fluid into a vein he felt considerably better. He had just survived an episode of diabetic ketoacidosis.

Bob made the classic mistake and could have died because of it. He had a minor viral gastroenteritis (tummy bug) which made him vomit. What he should have done as soon as he felt unwell was check his blood glucose. He should have taken his long-acting insulin regardless of whether he was vomiting or not and adjusted the dose of fast-acting insulin according to frequent blood glucose measurements. If necessary he could have had 2–6 units of fast-acting insulin every four hours. As it was he stopped his insulin at a time when his body needed it most.

Most illnesses increase the blood glucose because of increased resistance to insulin. Bob needed more insulin, not less. As he became increasingly insulin-deficient he started breaking down fats and making ketones. These made his blood acid and he started overbreathing to 'blow off' the acid. The very high glucose level caused severe polyuria and as he became more nauseated and iller he was less and less able to drink to replenish the lost fluid. *Never stop your insulin.*

Tony Tony is an engineer who has been diabetic for seven years. His diabetes was diagnosed when he had pneumonia and he had needed insulin injections at first. He lost weight and now manages to control his blood glucose on diet and glibenclamide pills, 10 mg with breakfast and 5 mg with lunch. He is now aged forty-nine.

Tony went to India last year and was thoroughly enjoying

himself when dysentery struck. He was miles away from a large town but had gone well prepared. He went to bed and drank large amounts of glucose and electrolyte solution made up with boiled water. Tony's blood glucose, which is usually between 4 and 8 mmol/l (72–144 mg/dl) rose to 22 mmol/l (396 mg/dl). He had had the foresight to ask his diabetes adviser to give him some soluble (regular) insulin to take with him and had discussed how to use it. Fortunately he had managed to keep it cool. He stopped taking his glibenclamide and started insulin injections – 10 units to start with and then adjusted the dose according to four-hourly blood glucose measurements.

After a gruelling four days the diarrhoea subsided and a thinner rather exhausted Tony restarted his glibenclamide (still checking his blood glucose regularly) and carried on with his journey.

Tony was familiar with both oral hypoglycaemic medication and insulin and had discussed potential problems with his diabetes adviser. He treated himself because he was miles from help. Had he been at home he would have contacted his doctor immediately. If you would like to learn how to use insulin to sort out your blood glucose when your oral hypoglycaemic pills are temporarily insufficient to control it ask your doctor if this would be possible. Make sure that you are absolutely clear about its use and the dosage regimen and do not allow the availability of insulin at home to delay your seeking help.

Sick days – general advice

Remember, if you feel ill, check your blood glucose frequently – at least four times a day. Never stop your insulin or oral hypoglycaemic pills. Consult your doctor if you have severe symptoms, are ill for more than a day, cannot control your blood glucose or are worried in any way. Doctors much prefer to be contacted early, when preventive measures can be taken, rather than too late, when a crisis has already occurred.

Ups and downs

Maggie Maggie is fifty-four years old and works as a personnel manager. She has had insulin-treated diabetes since she was forty-two and checks her blood-glucose meticulously. Maggie came for her annual check recently. 'I keep having to leave meetings to go to pass urine and I am so thirsty,' she said. I asked about her glucose control and she showed me the rows of values ranging from 11 to 17 mmol (198 to 306 mg/dl). She admitted that she had never been brave enough to alter her insulin 'in case something goes wrong'.

Most people can learn how to adjust their own treatment. Learn which insulin acts at what time of day and for how long. Ask your doctor to help you plan what to do if your blood glucose levels are too low or too high. If you are worried telephone your diabetes adviser to check that you are doing the right thing should the time come to alter your insulin. But please do not ignore high blood-glucose measurements.

Longer-term indicators of blood glucose concentration

A finger-prick blood sample tells you what your glucose is now. In clinics it is also possible to assess longer-term blood glucose concentration. This is done by taking advantage of a process called glycosylation – the linking of glucose to body proteins. The higher the blood glucose over the period in which the process occurs, the greater the concentration of glycosylated protein. Two measures are currently in use – haemoglobin Al_c and fructosamine. Fructosamine indicates the degree of hyperglycaemia over the past three weeks, haemoglobin Al_c is a longer-term measure covering the preceding four to six weeks.

Summary

- Aim for normal blood-glucose levels.
- Make sure that you prevent hypoglycaemia.
- If you become hypoglycaemic, eat glucose immediately. Learn to recognise symptoms early.
- Treat persistently high blood-glucose levels either by removing the cause or by altering diet, exercise, insulin or oral hypoglycaemic pills, or contact your doctor.
- *Never stop your insulin or pills.*
- *If in doubt ask for help earlier rather than later.*

9

Complications of diabetes

Diabetes may produce short-term symptoms arising from the high blood glucose concentrations. These soon settle with treatment by diet, exercise, insulin or pills. Over the years, though, some people with diabetes develop long-term symptoms due to diabetic tissue damage or complications. Some health care professionals may be reluctant to discuss tissue damage – 'We must not worry the patient.' However a person with diabetes can reduce the likelihood of developing tissue damage by careful attention to diet and health care. So you need to know about tissue damage so that you can work with your doctor to prevent it. If tissue damage does develop there are many helpful treatments; again, if you know what symptoms to look for you can seek help at a time when treatment can be most effective.

The following sections discuss each form of diabetic complication, factors influencing it, symptoms and signs and how it can be prevented and treated. Listed in this way it may look frightening. Remember, you are certainly not going to get all of these complications – if any. Most of you are healthy – the aim is to ensure that you stay that way.

Large and small blood-vessel damage

The two major forms of diabetic tissue damage are large (macro) and small (micro) blood-vessel disease (angiopathy). The medical names for these conditions are macroangiopathy and microangiopathy. Macroangiopathy may damage the large vessels supplying the heart, the legs and the brain as well as being linked with high blood pressure. Microangiopathy may damage the tiny blood vessels supplying the back of the eye, the kidney and the nerves and parts of the heart. Other processes, or a combination of factors, may damage nerves and feet and increase the risks of infection in people with diabetes.

The following sections describe each type of diabetic tissue damage, discuss how it can affect people and present ways of investigating and treating it. Researchers may disagree about the precise causes of diabetic complications – this is an enormous field of very active research – and different doctors may have very different ways of managing diabetic complications. Because I am writing for a large number of different readers I have had to generalise about some conditions and have tried to present the usual views about their management. Each of you is different and your doctor will be able to tell you what tests and treatment are most appropriate for you personally.

Many scientists have studied the causes of large- and small-vessel damage in diabetes. Some factors have emerged from several or many research studies as being more likely to lead to the development of new tissue damage or worsen existing tissue damage. You can alter many of these factors yourself and therefore reduce the risk of developing severe complications from diabetes.

Large blood-vessel disease (macroangiopathy)

Atherosclerosis

Atherosclerosis means furring up and hardening of the arteries. Most people in Western societies will have some evidence of atherosclerosis in their later years. If you have diabetes you are more likely than the general population to have heart disease, high blood pressure and narrowing of the arteries in the legs or brain – all related to atherosclerosis.

Arteries are the blood vessels which supply blood to every part of the body. Over the years fat is deposited in the lining of arteries. These deposits are called plaques. Calcium may also be deposited, making the plaques hard and brittle. Gradually the artery becomes narrowed and loses its elasticity. Clots may form on the plaques and can eventually block the artery. As the artery narrows, the part of the body it supplies receives less blood and is deprived of the oxygen and nutrients needed for functioning. This is called ischaemia. If the artery becomes blocked, the part it supplies will

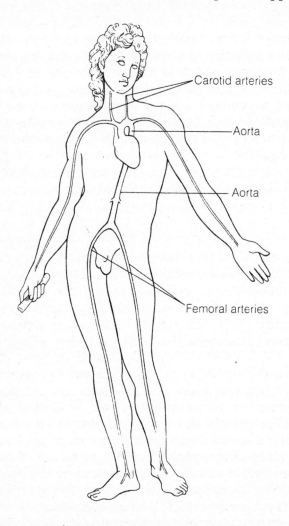

The main arteries in the body.

die. This is called infarction. Thus heart disease due to insufficient blood supply is called ischaemic heart disease, and permanent damage to the heart muscle (myocardium) from lack of blood supply is called myocardial infarction.

Risk factors for large blood-vessel disease (macroangiopathy)

If you smoke fifteen or more cigarettes a day you are at least eight times as likely to have severely narrowed leg arteries, causing pain on walking, as a non-smoker. Heavy smokers are about three times as likely to die from ischaemic heart disease as non-smokers. The more you smoke the more likely you are to die – not just from diseases of arteries but also from lung cancer. One in two smokers die from the complications of smoking. Smoking is so dangerous that it is worth giving up even at the expense of gaining weight, although it is obviously best if you manage to stay slim.

High blood fat levels

Two blood fats or lipids which should be checked regularly in people with diabetes are cholesterol and triglyceride. Total cholesterol should be below 5.2 mmol/l (200 mg/dl). It is made up of several lipoproteins (fatty proteins) – mainly high density lipoprotein (HDL), which exerts a protective effect upon blood vessels with a desirable level above 0.9 mmol/l (34 mg/dl), and low density lipoprotein (LDL), which is deposited in artery walls to produce atheromatous plaques. The desirable level for LDL varies according to your general state, but should probably be below 3.5 mmol/l (133 mg/dl) in people with diabetes. The triglyceride level should be under 2.3 mmol/l (87 mg/dl). In countries where the population has a high blood total cholesterol level there is a high death rate from ischaemic heart disease. The lower the cholesterol, the less the risk of dying from ischaemic heart disease. If you eat a diet high in saturated animal fats, you are more likely to have a high cholesterol than if you eat a low fat

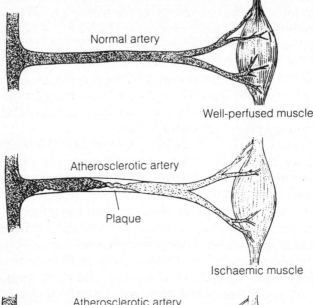

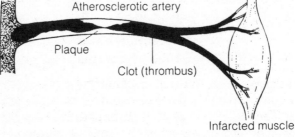

Atherosclerosis. The artery becomes partly blocked by deposits of plaque on which clots may develop, blocking the artery completely. The muscle first becomes damaged and then dies completely.

diet in which most fats are polyunsaturated vegetable products.

People with diabetes may have high cholesterol levels but are more likely to have raised triglyceride levels. This is because insulin is needed to break down triglyceride. High triglyceride levels may also increase the risk of ischaemic heart disease, especially with a low HDL cholesterol.

The first blood-fat lowering measure is to lose weight. This may be all that is needed to return the blood fats to normal. A high-fibre high-carbohydrate low-fat diet is the cornerstone of treatment. The percentage of the diet eaten as fats should be reduced to 25–30 per cent, with a high ratio of polyunsaturated: saturated fats. If you have a high blood cholesterol and/or triglyceride it is essential to modify your diet, but most doctors now recommend that we should all do this. People with high lipids should also stop drinking alcohol and maintain a normal blood glucose. Uncontrolled diabetes can cause very high triglyceride levels.

If your lipids remain too high despite good glucose balance and an appropriate diet, you will probably need lipid-lowering medication. This may include drugs called fibrates, which lower both cholesterol and triglyceride, or statins, whose main effect is cholesterol reduction. Most doctors would not give people over 70 years of age lipid-lowering drugs as their benefit above this age is not clear.

It is usually suggested that people with diabetes have their fasting blood lipid levels checked at least every three years, and some doctors would now advise annual checks.

High blood pressure

High blood pressure or hypertension can be a consequence of atherosclerosis but it may also worsen it. It is one of the major factors contributing to the development of ischaemic heart disease. The higher the systolic (pumped) blood pressure in men or women, the greater the rate of ischaemic heart disease. Thus, in men who entered one study aged forty to forty-nine years, approximately four out of five of those with systolic blood pressures of 180 mm Hg or more (see page 100) developed ischaemic heart disease during the next twenty-four years, compared with one in five of those with systolic blood pressures below 120 mm Hg. If you have high blood pressure you and your doctor must work at reducing it.

Overweight

Fat people are more likely to have a heart attack than slim people. This is probably due to the association of obesity with high blood pressure, cholesterol and glucose intolerance, although some people suggest that being fat is in itself a risk factor for heart disease. It is important to return to your ideal weight and stay there.

Lack of exercise

Exercise is hard to measure in a 'free range' population. Several studies have suggested that vigorous exercise taken regularly reduces the risk of myocardial infarction. This level of exercise is equivalent to running, skiing, swimming and tennis, for example. See page 39.

Glucose intolerance

Large studies have shown that the risk of having ischaemic heart disease is greater in people with impaired glucose tolerance (see page 10) in diabetes. People with definite diabetes are about twice as likely to die from myocardial infarction as those whose blood glucose is completely normal.

High blood-insulin concentrations

In non-diabetics high blood-insulin levels are associated with increased risk of atherosclerosis. There is some evidence from Oxford and Finland to suggest that heart disease in people with non-insulin-requiring diabetes may be linked with high insulin levels. This would suggest that it may be better to keep the glucose levels down with diet and exercise than with drugs which raise the blood insulin level.

Salt

Some authorities consider that a high salt (sodium chloride) intake raises the blood pressure. There has been some controversy over this but it seems reasonable to apply some commonsense. There is enough salt in our food for our bodies' needs without our adding more at the table.

Being a man

Middle-aged men are about six times as likely to die from a heart attack as middle-aged women. The women start to catch up when they stop having menstrual periods. However, once a woman develops diabetes she loses this hormonal protection. Diabetic women of all ages are as likely to have a heart attack as men.

Other factors

Even when one includes all the factors described, the greater risk of macroangiopathy in people with diabetes cannot be completely explained. One additional factor is that people with diabetes seem to have very 'sticky' blood, which clots easily. These clots may then take longer than usual to break down. Much research continues.

Small-vessel disease – microangiopathy

Large vessels – arteries – carry the blood from the heart to the major parts of the body. The arteries then divide into smaller and smaller tributaries until they become the fine capillaries which supply the cells themselves. In the eyes and kidneys of people with diabetes, capillary walls may thicken, reducing the exchange of nutrients and waste substances, or capillaries may become blocked by tiny clots. Some of the capillary walls become leaky.

The damage that this microvascular disease causes is called nephropathy in the kidney and retinopathy in the eye.

Risk factors for small-vessel disease

Duration of diabetes

The longer you have had diabetes, the more likely you are to have microvascular disease. Most people who have had diabetes for over twenty years have some evidence of retinopathy, although some people remain complication-free for much longer than this.

Age at onset of diabetes

This factor interacts with duration. Thus one in fourteen people under twenty years old when their diabetes was diagnosed will have retinopathy after ten years; one in four diagnosed diabetic when over forty will have retinopathy after ten years.

High blood glucose

There has long been evidence that people with high blood glucose levels are more likely to have small vessel complications than those with lower glucose levels. In 1993, the Diabetes Control and Complications Trial reported the results of a 9 year study of 1441 people with IDDM randomly allocated to conventional diabetes care or to very intensive blood glucose control. The intensive control group made frequent visits to their diabetes advisers with very careful treatment adjustment aiming to return the blood glucose to as near normal as safely possible. The main problem was avoiding hypoglycaemia.

The intensive control group had an average blood glucose level of 8.6 mmol/l (155 mg/dl) compared with 12.8 mmol/l (231 mg/dl) in the conventionally-treated group. Compared with the conventionally-treated group, the intensive control group reduced their risk of developing diabetic retinopathy by 76 per cent, and in those who already had retinopathy, its progression was slowed by 54 per cent. Intensive treatment reduced the appearance of obvious protein in the urine (a sign of diabetic kidney problems) by 54 per cent, and reduced the development of clinical neuropathy by 60 per cent.

We await the completion of the UK Prospective Diabetes Study of NIDDM but it is highly likely that this will show similar benefits from keeping the blood glucose near normal. In a previous Oxford project, we studied people who had had maturity-onset type diabetes for seven years. Those whose average fasting blood glucose was 14 mmol/l (252 mg/dl) or more were five times as likely to have retinopathy as those with normal glucose levels.

Hypertension

High blood pressure is a risk factor for both diabetic and non-diabetic kidney disease. If you already have nephropathy, keeping the blood pressure normal slows the progression of kidney damage considerably. Hypertension probably increases the risk of developing new retinopathy and worsens existing retinopathy.

Obesity

Some studies have suggested that obesity increases the likelihood of having microangiopathy.

Heredity

Some diabetic families seem remarkably free from microangiopathy. Other families with a strong history of diabetes also seem to have a strong history of microangiopathy, especially retinopathy. If you belong to a family like this, you should have your eyes checked more often than other people and reduce other risk factors.

Other factors

Other research suggests that glycosylation of proteins (remember haemoglobin Al_c, page 80) may be involved in the development of some tissue damage.

Summary

- Some people with diabetes develop tissue damage over the years.
- People with diabetes are more likely to develop

macroangiopathy or large blood-vessel disease than non-diabetics. You can reduce this excess risk by not smoking, keeping your weight down, controlling your blood fat and glucose levels, keeping your blood pressure normal and exercising regularly.

- Small vessel disease or microangiopathy occurs only in diabetes. You can reduce the risk of developing small vessel disease by controlling your blood glucose and blood pressure and keeping your weight within normal limits.

10

Large blood-vessel disease

This chapter looks at macroangiopathy or large blood-vessel disease – ischaemic heart disease, hypertension, peripheral vascular disease and cerebrovascular disease. People with diabetes are more likely to suffer from all these diseases than non-diabetics.

Heart disease

The heart is a muscle which works as a pump. All muscles need a good blood supply to deliver oxygen and nutrients and remove waste substances. At rest the heart muscle (myocardium) needs a small blood flow. When you are exercising and all the other muscles in the body require more blood, your heart has to work harder to deliver it to them. Your heart muscle therefore needs more blood too. The blood is supplied to the heart muscle by the coronary arteries.

If a coronary artery becomes narrowed by atherosclerosis the area of muscle it serves gets less blood. This process is called ischaemic heart disease. As the narrowing of the coronary artery worsens, the muscle becomes seriously deprived of blood (ischaemic), especially at times when the heart is working hard, e.g. during exercise or excitement. The resulting lack of oxygen and build up of waste substances produces pain – called angina pectoris. If the coronary artery becomes completely blocked by plaque or a clot (thrombus) the muscle eventually dies – myocardial infarction. This event is also called a coronary thrombosis. People with diabetes may also have small blood-vessel damage within heart muscle, reducing its function.

Symptoms of heart disease

Many people with mild coronary artery disease never have symptoms from it. Do not imagine symptoms.

Chest pain

Central, crushing or tight chest-pain sometimes radiating down the arms or up into the neck is called angina pectoris. Classically it occurs with exertion or stress and is relieved by rest or by glyceryl trinitrate tablets or spray under the tongue. This medication should work within ten minutes. If the pain is very severe, frightening or prolonged, or fails to respond to rest or nitrates, it may be due to myocardial infarction rather than angina, so call an ambulance immediately. While you are waiting for help to arrive, chew an

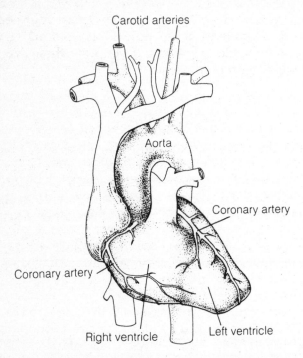

The heart, showing the major arteries leaving it and the coronary arteries which supply the heart itself.

aspirin – it will help your heart. (Obviously people who are allergic to aspirin should avoid it.)

Most of us get twinges of pain the chest from time to time, usually due to harmless muscle spasms (medical students are prone to this and always imagine the worst). Most chest pains are not heart pain, but if you have new, persistent or severe pains consult your doctor.

Breathlessness

Many conditions produce shortness of breath on exertion. One cause is weakness of the heart muscle, for example due to previous myocardial infarction. The technical term is left-ventricular failure. Shortness of breath when lying flat or sudden lack of breath in the night, especially if associated with a cough with frothy white sputum is usually due to left-ventricular failure. Heart failure does not mean your heart has stopped completely – it just means it is not working as efficiently as it should at present. If you have these symptoms, for whatever reason, see your doctor.

Ankle swelling

Puffiness of the ankles, especially towards evening, which pits when you press it with a finger is called ankle oedema. Many of us have this in very hot weather or if we have been on our feet all day. If it is severe or persistent it may be a sign of right-ventricular failure, also called congestive cardiac failure. Again, this is due to the reduced pumping power of the heart muscle – a different bit of the heart this time. However, there are also many other causes of ankle swelling.

Palpitations

This is an awareness of abnormally fast or uneven beating of the heart; for example, after drinking too much tea and coffee. It is rarely a serious symptom but if it makes you feel ill when it happens, or keeps happening, see your doctor.

What may happen when you see the doctor

Story and examination

First, your doctor will want a clear story of your symptoms, in the order in which they happened if possible. Write this down beforehand if you think you may forget something. Then he will examine you fully, checking the pulses and blood pressure, feeling the heart impulse, listening to the heart sounds, and checking for congestion in the lungs, liver and ankles.

Tests

Your doctor will probably order an electrocardiogram – an ECG or EKG. This is a recording of the electrical forces which stimulate your heart to beat. These electrical impulses spread rhythmically throughout the heart muscle. The different patterns on the ECG trace can show if a part of the heart is being deprived of oxygen or has been permanently damaged. However, the ECG can be normal between attacks of angina, so your doctor may request an exercise ECG so that he can look at the electrical recording while you walk on a treadmill.

If the ECGs show areas of heart muscle which are being deprived of blood, some medical centres will go on to do coronary angiograms – special X-rays which detect dye injected into the coronary arteries through a tube passed up through a tiny hole in a groin artery.

Echocardiography uses an ultrasound probe run gently over the skin (as in examining unborn babies in the womb) to produce an image of the heart. Other tests may involve the use of radioactive tracers, concentrated briefly in the heart, which allow measurement of how the heart is working. A simple test which shows heart size and evidence of left-ventricular failure is a chest X-ray.

Blood tests may include glucose and haemoglobin Al_c to check on glucose balance, fasting blood cholesterol and triglyceride concentration and 'cardiac' enzymes. These enzymes are chemicals released by dying heart muscle in myocardial infarction.

Myocardial infarction

If you have ECG changes and an increase in cardiac enzyme levels, with or without a history of chest pain, your doctor will diagnose a myocardial infarct. You will usually be admitted to hospital for treatment, rest and monitoring. Clot-busting treatment (thrombolysis) dissolves the clot in the coronary artery. The sooner thrombolytic treatment is given the better – so make sure you get to hospital quickly. You will then spend the first few days in bed and then gradually get back on your feet. Most people stay in hospital for one to two weeks and spend four to six weeks gradually becoming mobile again at home. People who have had a myocardial infarct can usually expect to be back working within three months. You should not drive for two months. Be guided by your doctor about increasing your exercise and returning to work.

Many people have no further heart trouble – especially if they avoid risk factors. Stop smoking, check your diet (especially the fat content) and watch your blood pressure. Your blood glucose will probably rise, so do not be surprised if you need insulin treatment while you are in hospital. You will probably need to take aspirin long-term and probably a beta blocker (see page 102) or ACE inhibitor (see page 103) to protect the heart.

Angina pectoris

Brief episodes of chest pain brought on by exertion or stress and relieved by rest or nitrates, with or without ECG change, may lead your doctor to a diagnosis of angina. If you are having frequent episodes your doctor may advise rest until your treatment has been sorted out.

The first thing to do is go over the risk factor list. Which ones apply to you. Do you smoke? Are you fat? What about blood fats and blood pressure? Do something about them immediately, after discussion with your doctor. Most people with angina can exercise safely until stopped by their chest pain, but check with your doctor before starting an exercise programme.

There are several drugs to treat angina.

Nitrates

Initial medication will probably be glyceryl trinitrate tablets dissolved under the tongue or an equivalent nitrate spray. There are other slower-acting forms of nitrates; these may come as pills or as patches to be applied to the skin.

Nitrates help open up or dilate blood vessels all over the body, including the heart; they can thus help in the treatment of heart failure. If you use skin patches, do not inject insulin near a patch – dilated blood vessels will absorb it too quickly. Nitrates may make people flushed and cause headaches.

Beta blockers

These pills help angina by slowing down the rate of the heart and reducing its work-load. They also lower the blood pressure. There is a huge range of such drugs – propranolol, oxprenolol, metoprolol, atenolol are some of the common ones. Notice that they all end in -olol. Older forms, like propranolol, are called non-selective – they act all over the body, not just on the heart and blood vessels. They may provoke asthma in susceptible people and also reduce your warning of hypoglycaemia by suppressing adrenaline (epinephrine) release.

If people whose diabetes is treated by insulin or oral hypoglycaemic pills need a beta blocker it should be a selective one (note that even selective beta blockers may cause asthma or reduce hypoglycaemia warning). All beta blockers can control the heart rhythm, but they may worsen heart failure in some circumstances and may raise the blood glucose. They may cause bad dreams, muscle fatigue and tiredness. These effects tend to improve with time.

Calcium antagonists

Calcium antagonists reduce the oxygen demand by the heart muscle. Ones used in Britain are called nifedipine, nicardipine, diltiazam and verapamil. They can cause flushing and occasionally heart failure in certain people. Some may be helpful in steadying the heart rhythm, as are beta blockers.

Reducing risk factors

None of these medications will be of much use if you do not pay attention to reducing your risk factors. Stop smoking, check your weight and your diet, watch your blood fats and your blood pressure and take treatment for them if necessary. Most people with angina can return to work and enjoy life.

Surgery

In some people a pill treatment is not wholly effective and they may be helped by coronary-artery bypass surgery. This is an operation in which the narrowed coronary arteries are bypassed by lengths of vein taken from your leg. Coronary-artery bypass is also offered to people with narrowings at critical parts of the coronary arterial system. It is also possible to open the narrowing by inflating a tiny balloon inside the artery – coronary angioplasty.

Heart disease – summary

- People with diabetes are more likely to develop heart disease than non-diabetics.
- Stop smoking, eat the right diet, keep blood fats and blood pressure normal, take regular exercise; these help to prevent heart disease.
- Prompt attention to the warning symptoms can allow treatment to help minimise further trouble.

High blood pressure or hypertension

People with newly-diagnosed diabetes have higher blood pressures than non-diabetics. People with established diabetes are also prone to hypertension – one American study suggested a 50 per cent greater prevalence compared with non-diabetics.

What is hypertension?

Every time your heart beats, the heart muscle pumps a spurt of blood into the arteries and around the body. The pumping pressure measured in the artery in the arm is called the systolic blood pressure. The resting pressure, between heart beats, is called the diastolic blood pressure. The pressures are measured in millimetres of mercury (mm Hg) up the column of a sphygmomanometer or blood-pressure machine.

It is difficult to define normal limits because blood pressure varies with age and from minute to minute, and measurement techniques also vary. The upper limit of normal blood pressure is regarded as about 160 mm Hg systolic and 90 mm Hg diastolic, usually written as 160/90. The higher the blood pressure, the greater the risk of ischaemic heart disease, heart failure, stroke and kidney disease, whether you are diabetic or not.

The level at which one starts treating high blood pressure has been the subject of much controversy. Most doctors would treat someone with diastolic pressures of 100 mm Hg or above. Treatment of diastolic pressures of 90–100 mm Hg is more debatable, although there is evidence that this reduces complications of hypertension. Levels of systolic pressure that should be treated have not been clearly defined, yet it is this that is linked with ischaemic heart disease. I would be worried if a person consistently had systolic pressures over 180 mm Hg.

The vast majority of people with high blood pressure are completely unaware of it. Headaches are rarely a symptom of hypertension – but they do prompt doctors to measure the blood pressure!

What your doctor may do

When you see a doctor ask him to measure your blood pressure. Hypertension is a treatable condition and its complications can be prevented. If he finds that you have hypertension he will probably remeasure it several times to check. But do not wait for the verdict – look at the risk factors on pages 85–89 immediately and see what you can do to help yourself.

If your blood pressure is definitely elevated, then your doctor will check your pulses, heart, lungs, eyes (for signs of blood-pressure change in the eye arteries) and kidneys. He may also check for the rare causes of hypertension (e.g. hormone abnormalities). Most people have so-called essential hypertension – no obvious cause is found.

Tests

These include blood electrolytes, urea and creatinine (to check kidney function) and fasting fats. The doctor will check your urine for cells, protein and infection, and he will arrange an ECG and chest X-ray, looking for heart enlargement or failure. He may order an ultrasound kidney scan, or an intravenous urogram – a kidney X-ray in which dye injected into an arm vein is concentrated in the kidneys and outlines their shape and that of the urinary tract. You may be asked to save your urine for 24 hrs to check steroid or adrenaline excretion or to monitor creatinine clearance.

Treatment of hypertension

Risk factors

Smoking, obesity, high blood fats and possibly eating too much salt all put you at risk. Check these immmediately. Any one of the risk factors increases the damage from blood pressure.

Relaxation

Easy to say, hard to do. Stress raises blood pressure; full relaxation lowers it. Try to reduce stress at work and home. Another book in this series, *Stress and Relaxation* by Jane Madders, will help you.

Pills

There are over forty blood-pressure lowering pills listed in the *British National Formulary*. This means that it is possible to find one that suits you. This is important. You and your blood-pressure pills will be together for the rest of your life – it is unusual for someone with hypertension to stop needing treatment. Don't think because your blood pressure is normal you can stop your pills. It is normal *because of* your pills.

Diuretics

Diuretics promote urinary fluid loss and probably lower blood pressure by reducing blood volume. They include thiazides, frusemide and bumetanide. Diuretics may raise the blood glucose and uric acid (occasionally causing gout) and lower the blood potassium level.

Spironolactone and amiloride are different diuretics which do not cause potassium loss. In men spironolactone may induce breast fullness.

Beta blockers

See page 98. They are very effective at lowering the blood pressure, although again it is unclear exactly how they work. They are widely used and each doctor has one or two he prefers. Long-acting selective ones, like atenolol, with a once-daily dose are popular. Do not stop them abruptly – you may get palpitations.

Vasodilators

If you widen (dilate) blood vessels the resistance to the heart's pumping acting is less, which means that the blood pressure falls. Nitrates, nifedipine and verapamil (discussed on pages 98–99) are vasodilators; others are hydrallazine and prazosin. All of these drugs may make you flushed. They can also make the blood pressure fall when you stand up (normally the blood pressure increases briefly when you stand, in order to compensate for gravity). This postural hypotension may make you dizzy or faint.

ACE inhibitors

These drugs block hormones which raise blood pressure. ACE inhibitors should be started cautiously as some people are very sensitive to them. Their effect may be increased if the patient is already taking diuretics. They may be particularly helpful in treating hypertension in diabetes. Some ACE inhibitors are captopril, enalapril, lisinopril and perindopril.

Others

Some drugs act on the nervous system to reset the controls on the blood pressure throughout the body. Methyl-dopa is a very effective anti-hypertensive, less popular nowadays because it can cause drowsiness, depression and impotence. Clonidine is a similar drug also used to treat migraine and menopausal symptoms. If you are on clonidine you must not stop it suddenly or your blood pressure will rebound – rise rapidly – and you may have a stroke.

Rules for anti-hypertensive pills

- Know which pills you are taking, how they work and what their hazards (if any) are.
- Take them until your doctor tells you to stop.
- If they upset you, tell your doctor immediately.
- Never stop clonidine or beta blockers abruptly.
- Remember that these pills may have an effect on your diabetes, and that they could interact with other pills – so always tell a new doctor what you are taking.

Josephine is seventy-three years old. She has high blood pressure as well as diabetes, and obtains her pills on repeat prescription forms. In diabetic clinic she complained of giddiness every time she got up in the morning and if she stood up suddenly. Her blood pressure was 110/70 falling to 80/50 on standing. I asked about her medication and she produced a bag of pill bottles. 'The doctor gave me some new ones,' she said, producing bottles of atenolol and hydrochlorthdiazide. 'These are the old ones. I still take them every day.' Bottles of propranolol and bendrofluazide appeared. Josephine had no idea what her pills were called or what they did. She had forgotten that her doctor had told her to stop the old pills and was taking two beta blockers and two thiazides religously. Small wonder that her blood pressure was very low and fell every time she stood up.

Self-monitoring

You can buy your own sphygmomanometer to monitor your blood pressure at home. Ask your doctor about this. There are several machines to choose from – these which pump up the cuff for you are best (if you pump air into the cuff yourself it may raise your blood pressure.)

Hypertension – summary

- High blood pressure is common in diabetics.
- People rarely have any symptoms of a high blood pressure.
- Blood pressure should be checked regularly. Consider self-monitoring.
- If you have high blood pressure, check your weight and slim if necessary, stop smoking, avoid salt and ask your doctor to check your blood fat levels.
- Reduce stress and learn how to relax.
- Take your anti-hypertensive pills precisely as recommended by your doctor.
- Do not worry about blood pressure. High blood pressure can be controlled with treatment.

Peripheral vascular disease

This means disease of the arteries supplying the limbs. People with diabetes are at least three times more likely to have symptomatic peripheral vascular disease than non-diabetics. Mild peripheral vascular disease is usually symptomless, but may give rise to the following.

Pain in the legs

Tight pain in the calves, thighs or buttocks, which comes on while walking and settles rapidly with rest, is called intermittent claudication (intermittent limping). If the arteries are severely narrowed there may even be pain in the feet at rest.

Cold feet

Cold feet, white on elevation and often purple/red after standing or sitting for a long time, with reduced hair growth on the lower legs, all suggest poor circulation.

Black toes

This occurs when the blood supply to these toes is blocked, and indicates gangrene. Contact your doctor immediately.

What your doctor may do

He will discuss your symptoms with you and examine all the pulses throughout your body, including neck and groins. He will check your blood pressure, heart and eyes and feel your abdomen to check the aorta.

Tests

He will take detailed measurements of your pulses with an ultrasound probe run gently over the skin above the position of the pulses. He will check your fasting blood fats, and ECG.

If it seems that a major artery is severely narrowed the doctor may order femoral angiograms – a tube is threaded into the artery through a puncture in the groin under local anaesthetic and X-rays are taken as the dye flows down the arteries.

Treatment of peripheral vascular disease

Avoidance of risk factors

Over 90 per cent of people with peripheral vascular disease smoke. If you smoke, stop immediately – every cigarette you smoke does a little more damage to your arteries. Ask your doctor about your blood fats and take your anti-hypertensive pills if you have high blood pressure. (NB Beta blockers may worsen intermittent claudication.)

Exercise

Keep going if possible, and walk as far as you can several times a day to encourage an alternative circulation to develop. Intermittent claudication may resolve itself spontaneously.

Protect your feet

The circulation may be very poor in cold weather; wear warm socks and check feet frequently in winter. Poor circulation also means that injuries and infections take longer to heal.

Vasodilators

These are rarely helpful as they cannot dilate atherosclerotic arteries.

Peripheral activators

Naftidofuryl oxalate improves utilisation of oxygen and glucose and can ease symptoms of peripheral vascular disease.

Surgery

It may be possible to bypass a narrowed or blocked artery using a tube of artificial material. Sometimes the plaque can be cleared or the narrowed artery widened. However, the effort will be wasted if you carry on smoking.

Peripheral vascular disease – summary

- Peripheral vascular disease is commoner in diabetics than in non-diabetics.
- It may cause pain in the legs on walking, cold feet and, rarely, pain at rest or gangrenous toes.
- *Stop smoking immediately.* Check blood fats and blood pressure.
- Walk regularly and look after your feet. Keep them warm in winter.

Cerebrovascular disease

This is disease of the arteries supplying the brain. The main arteries to the brain are the carotids on each side of the neck. There are also vertebral arteries running up the spinal column.

Symptoms of cerebrovascular disease

Most mature Westerners have minor degrees of cerebrovascular atherosclerosis – it does not noticeably affect their brain function. Symptoms are extremely variable and depend on which area of brain has been deprived of its blood supply. These are some of the commoner symptoms.

Weakness or clumsiness of an arm or leg

Sudden loss of power in an arm and leg on one side – a stroke – may be the first sign of cerebrovascular disease. It can be transient or permanent (although some improvement nearly always occurs).

Loss of sensation

Sudden loss of sensation may be due to cerebrovascular disease, but diabetic neuropathy is a commoner cause.

Difficulty with speech

There may be difficulty in finding what you want to say or in getting the words out. This is called dysphasia.

Confusion or poor memory

Diffuse cerebrovascular disease can cause someone to become muddled or forgetful.

Loss of consciousness

In a severe stroke the person may be unconscious.

Severe dizziness, vertigo and drop attacks

These are common symptoms and rarely serious. They may indicate cerebrovascular disease or atherosclerosis in the vertebral arteries. There are many other causes of dizziness, including arthritis in the neck, low blood pressure on standing and ear diseases.

What your doctor may do

This obviously depends on how ill you are. The doctor will want to know the sequence of events as this is very important in diagnosing the problem. He will examine your pulse, blood pressure, heart, neck arteries, eyes, face, arms and legs, including muscle movement and strength, reflexes, coordination and sensation.

Tests

The doctor will check your glucose, haemoglobin Al$_c$ and fasting blood fats levels and run an ECG. Sometimes a computerised tomogram will be performed (CT scan); this shows which area of the brain has been affected and what has happened – a plain skull X-ray is of little help. An ultrasound scan may detect narrowing of the carotid arteries. If a narrowing of a surgically-accessible artery is suspected, a carotid angiogram X-ray may be performed; dye is injected into the carotid artery and rapid pictures taken as it flows through the brain arteries.

Stroke and transient ischaemic attacks

A stroke is the ordinary term for any episode of impaired brain function because its blood supply is blocked or a blood vessel has burst. The technical terms are cerebral thrombosis (clot arising in a brain artery), cerebral embolus (clot from somewhere else lodging in a brain artery) and cerebral haemorrhage (a bleed into the brain). People with diabetes are about twice as likely to have a stroke as non-diabetics.

A transient ischaemic attack is a temporary stroke lasting for less than twenty-four hours and leaving no permanent damage. It is due to part of the brain being briefly deprived of oxygen.

Minor strokes are fairly common and rarely cause much disturbance of function. In the more severe, and fortunately rarer, sort of stroke the person loses consciousness for a few hours. On waking he cannot move the arm and leg on one side of the body, and speech may be difficult. The person may have difficulty eating initially, and choke easily. Over the next day or two power starts to return to the limbs and the speech and eating begin to improve. The process of recovery begins.

Treatment of cerebrovascular disease

- Avoidance of risk factors (see pages 85–89). Blood pressure may go up during a stroke and long-term hypertension needs treating.
- Care of the unconscious person, keeping their airway clear.

- Physiotherapy, speech therapy and occupational therapy. The exercises should be performed as often as possible and family members should learn how to help.
- In cases of cerebral thrombosis or embolus, doctors may recommend aspirin or anticoagulants. Aspirin treatment can be particularly helpful in transient ischaemic attacks.
- In some cases, surgical widening and 'defurring' of narrowed carotid arteries may reduce the likelihood of further transient ischaemic attacks or strokes.
- Control blood glucose; it goes up even if you are not eating.
- It is easy to become depressed after a stroke. Family and friends should provide a lot of comfort and encouragement.

Cerebrovascular disease – summary

- People with diabetes are more likely to have a stroke than non-diabetics.
- You may have no symptoms of cerebrovascular disease. Symptoms depend on which part of the brain has had insufficient blood supply.
- Most people who have strokes recover and get back to normal.
- Do exercises prescribed; watch your weight, blood pressure and blood fats; do not smoke.
- Keep cheerful.

Summary – macrovascular disease

- People with diabetes are more likely to have ischaemic heart disease, hypertension, peripheral vascular disease and cerebrovascular disease than non-diabetics.
- It is possible to prevent or considerably reduce the risk of developing these complications.

- Do not smoke.
- Eat a high-fibre low-fat diet. Keep within your ideal body weight. Reduce salt.
- Check your fasting blood cholesterol and triglyceride levels once a year (more if raised).
- Exercise regularly and build up to vigorous exercise (be guided by your doctor).
- Learn to relax.
- Do not imagine symptoms – most of you are well and will remain so. If you do experience any of the symptoms described, see your doctor immediately. If he prescribes medication take it carefully in full knowledge of what you are taking, what it does and its side effects.

11

Eye problems

Diabetes can affect the eyes in several ways. Diabetic retinopathy occurs only in diabetes and is due to microangiopathy. However, people with diabetes are also more prone to cataract and other eye problems than the general population. Squints occur occasionally.

Symptoms of diabetic eye disease

None

Most people have no symptoms of early diabetic eye disease. That is why it is vital for an expert to check your eyes annually.

Blurred vision

This is usually linked with high blood glucose concentrations and settles within a few weeks of the glucose returning to normal. Tell your doctor.

Reduced visual acuity

If you cannot read as well or see as far or as accurately as before, get your eyes checked.

Loss of vision

If you lose any part of your vision see your doctor the same day.

Painful or red eye

This is unlikely to be related to diabetic eye trouble, but needs investigating anyway. Occasionally people with diabetes develop glaucoma – raised pressure in the eye – and this can be painful.

Double vision

Diabetic nerve damage may weaken eye muscles causing double vision.

'I need new glasses'

Perhaps. But never buy new glasses until you have had your eyes checked by your diabetes doctor and/or an ophthalmologist – the visual difficulty may be temporary.

What your doctor may do

He will discuss your story with you; the sequence of events may be particularly helpful here. Was it a sudden visual loss or gradual blurring? He will measure your visual acuity and check your eye movements if necessary.

Unless he suspects you have glaucoma, he will put dilating drops in your eyes to make the pupils larger (nowadays these wear off quickly or can be reversed by other drops). When the drops have worked he will examine first the lens then the retina (the light-sensitive film at the back of the eye) with a magnifying torch or ophthalmoscope. This examination should be carried out every year, regardless of whether you have any symptoms.

Tests

He will check your blood glucose control. If you have retinopathy you may have a fluoroscein angiogram. Yellow dye injected into an arm vein shows up retinal vessels which are then photographed. It occasionally makes people feel nauseous and may make you yellow for a few days but it is not painful. Blood tests will include those for glucose and haemoglobin Al$_c$.

Diabetic retinopathy

The retina is the light-sensitive film at the back of the eye which transmits visual signals to the brain. The earliest changes in diabetes are miniature capillary blow-outs called micro-aneurysms. Small bleeds may occur forming dot-and-blot haemorrhages. Fatty exudates leak through the capillary walls; if the exudates cover the area of best vision, or macula, sight will be impaired. All these changes are called background retinopathy.

As the capillary tissue damage continues, areas of the retina are deprived of their blood supply. They release a factor which stimulates growth of new vessels. Unfortunately these new vessels grow forwards into the clear (vitreous) jelly through which we see, and are very fragile. They may tear, in which case blood pours out into the jelly, blocking out the view. This is called a vitreous haemorrhage.

The development of new vessels signals proliferative retinopathy – a more serious but much rarer condition than background retinopathy. The damaged retina can also swell. If this occurs at the macula, vision deteriorates. Severe visual loss or blindness from diabetic retinopathy is uncommon.

Treatment of diabetic retinopathy

Risk factors

Gradually return your blood glucose to normal; over-rapid normalisation of the blood glucose may temporarily worsen retinopathy. Have your blood pressure checked.

Laser or xenon-arc photocoagulation

This is used to destroy areas of damaged retina which can stimulate new vessel growth. Photocoagulation can seal leaking microaneurysms and the new vessels. Treatment may be spread over days or weeks. Laser photocoagulatiaon is carried out as an out-patient procedure using local anaesthetic eye drops. Xenon-arc photocoagulation is given with an injection of local anaesthetic under the eye or under general anaesthetic. In both cases dilating drops are used and vision will be blurred with increased sensitivity to light for several hours after treatment. You should not exercise vigorously for several weeks after treatment (ask your ophthalmologist about this). The treatment may reduce your peripheral vision (the edges of your field of view).

Martin is a successful farmer and is now aged forty-four years. At the age of twenty-eight diabetes was diagnosed. His symptoms were easily controlled on diet and insulin treatment as he continued to build up his farm. Gradually he started missing his diabetic clinic appointments and eventually he stopped attending altogether. He felt all right and it seemed a long way to come for a routine check. It was ten years since his last visit when I saw him at a clinic to convert patients from U40 insulin to U100 strength. He is a well-tanned healthy-looking man and denied any diabetic symptoms. He said he never tested his urine for glucose and never altered his insulin dose.

When I examined his eyes I was horrified. He had proliferative retinopathy in both, with fronds of new vessels spreading forwards into the vitreous jelly. I sent him straight to the eye hospital where they started photocoagulation treatment. Fortunately the new vessels regressed. Martin now has regular diabetes and eye check-ups.

Cataract

Cataracts are due to desposition of opaque substances in the lens of the eye. This impairs vision, just as a dirty camera lens spoils your photographs. Several Americn studies found cataracts in about one in six diabetics over fifty years old but only in about one in ten non-diabetics.

People with newly-diagnosed diabetes may have temporary cataracts. As you grow older you are more likely to develop cataracts anyway, but this process happens at an earlier age in diabetes.

The only treatment at present is to remove the lens containing the cataract. Sometimes lens implants can be inserted at or after this operation. For most people a change of glasses will be needed afterwards.

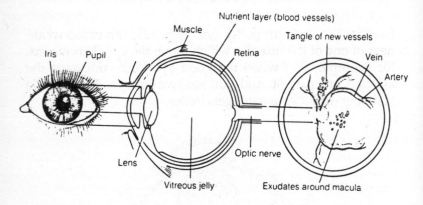

In the centre is a vertical section through a normal eye, while on the right is what the doctor sees when he looks through the pupil of someone with severe diabetic retinopathy.

Annie is seventy-three and lives in an old-persons' community. Her vision had been deteriorating for several years and it saddened her because she had not been able to see her little grandson properly. She was convinced she would never see again.

For about six months she had drunk twenty cups of tea a day and been passing a lot of urine. Her family doctor found her to have diabetes and also severe cataracts. He treated the diabetes and referred her to an eye surgeon. She had a cataract removed three months ago and got her new glasses just in time to see her new baby grand-daughter. She is delighted they are christening her Ann.

Retinal arterial or venous blockage

These conditions are uncommon. Retinal vein thrombosis is more likely to occur in people with diabetes, hypertension or high blood-fat levels. It may be followed by proliferative retinopathy. Retinal arteries can also become blocked, causing visual loss and areas of retinal ischaemia.

Disorders of eye movement

Rarely diabetic neuropathy (see page 125) can cause weakness of one of the muscles which move the eye. This means, for example, that when the good eye looks sideways the affected one cannot, and you see two images. This double vision or diplopia usually gets better.

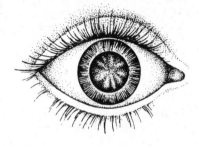

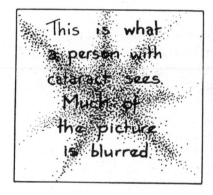

Cataracts develop in the lens of the eye, so that the light cannot enter the eye so effectively. The diagram demonstrates the sort of image someone with cataracts receives.

Summary

- Background diabetic retinopathy is common, proliferative retinopathy is rare. Both types are preventable and treatable.
- Cataract and glaucoma are commoner in people with diabetes than non-diabetics. They can be treated.
- Contact your doctor immediately if you notice any deterioration in your vision or have any other problems with your eyes.
- Keep your blood glucose normal and take any anti-hypertensive pills as prescribed.
- Have your eyes checked once a year.

12

Kidney and urinary tract problems

Urine removes excess fluid and waste substances from the body. Urine is made in the kidneys and passes down the ureters to collect in the urinary bladder in the pelvis. From the bladder the urine is voided from the body through the urethra.

Whereas doctors can see retinopathy on examination, kidney disease can be detected only if it causes changes in the urine (for example protein in the urine) or in blood tests, or if it produces symptoms.

Symptoms

You may be unaware that your kidney function is deteriorating until the damage is severe. This is why it is important that you or your doctor checks your kidney function regularly.

Pain passing urine

Dysuria or stinging or burning pain as you pass your urine may be a sign of urine infection.

Urinary frequency

Urine infection also causes the desire to pass small volumes of urine very frequently.

Polyuria and nocturia

In diabetes the commonest reason for passing lots of urine frequently (including night-time) is high blood-glucose levels. If your glucose is normal, you are not over-drinking and you have polyuria your kidneys may not be concentrating urine properly.

Abnormal urine

Smelly, cloudy urine is a sign of infection. Blood in the urine (haematuria) should be reported to your doctor straightaway unless it is due to menstruation (a period).

Loin pain

Pain in the back below the ribs or in the sides may be due to kidney infection.

Difficulty with urination, frequency, nocturia

These are all symptoms of an enlarged prostate – nothing to do with diabetes, but common in men over forty.

What your doctor may do

He will listen to your symptoms and examine you generally, especially your blood pressure, eyes (retinopathy and nephropathy usually occur together), abdomen and pelvic organs.

Tests

Examination of the urine is very important, so be prepared to give a specimen. Urine will be checked for blood, protein and pus cells, and cultured for bacterial infection. Other microscopic abnormalities may give clues to kidney disease.

Blood tests include glucose balance, electrolytes, urea, creatinine, calcium, phosphate, albumin and urate. You may need to collect all your urine for a twenty-four-hour period to measure protein output or creatinine clearance – an indicator of kidney function. Further tests are a kidney ultrasound and an intravenous urogram (see page 101).

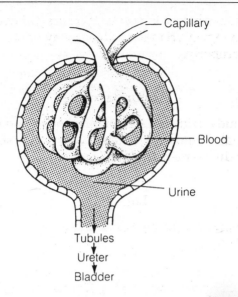

Capillary

Blood

Urine

Tubules
Ureter
Bladder

A glomerulus in the kidney. Waste substances are filtered out of the blood in the knot of capillaries and eventually pass out of the body in the urine. Each kidney contains many million glomeruli.

Diabetic nephropathy

In the kidney waste substances are filtered from the blood through tangles of capillaries called glomeruli and collected into tiny tubes. The waste substances and water flow into larger tubes and eventually down the ureters into the bladder. In diabetes the membrane around the capillaries may thicken, preventing the passage of wastes. Gradually the glomeruli solidify and die. You have two kidneys and millions of glomeruli, so it takes years for the loss of glomeruli to make a noticeable difference to kidney function.

The earliest sign of damage is usually the leakage of tiny amounts of protein into the urine – microalbuminuria. Both this, and larger amounts (albuminuria) can be detected by dipstick testing. American and European studies showed that one in eight people with diabetes had proteinuria. If you have proteinuria you should have a thorough kidney check –

the protein may not be due to diabetes but infection, for example.

If kidney damage progesses, the kidneys start to fail. Waste substances are no longer filtered from the blood and start to accumulate, as may water, producing ankle swelling, shortness of breath, weakness, itchy skin, tiredness, anaemia.

Treatment of diabetic nephropathy

Avoidance of risk factors

The most important of these is high blood pressure. Untreated hypertension rapidly worsens diabetic nephropathy, so it is vital to return the blood pressure to normal and keep it there. Good blood glucose control is also essential. Return your blood glucose to normal and keep it there. One practical point is that insulin requirements will fall as the kidneys fail and you may have unexpected hypoglycaemic attacks. Do not smoke.

Avoidance of infection

Wash between your legs every day. Learn the symptoms of urinary infection. If your doctor agrees, keep a urine specimen pot and antibiotics at home to start treatment immediately. First send a midstream urine sample to your doctor.

Diet

To start with, the ordinary diabetic diet will help to keep your blood glucose controlled, while plenty of fluids will help keep the urinary tract flushed through. However, if you have any evidence of kidney damage, you may be advised to avoid salt and restrict protein and fluids.

Diuretics

If you start accumulating fluids, your doctor may start you on these – frusemide and bumetanide are two common ones.

Mineral and vitamin supplements

These may be needed, depending on the type of kidney failure.

Dialysis and transplants

If the kidney failure worsens you may need dialysis – artificial filtering of the waste substances from the blood. This may be haemodialysis, in which your blood is filtered on a machine. Another form is continuous ambulatory peritoneal dialysis, in which fluid is run into the abdominal cavity where it absorbs all the wastes and is then run out again. At this point your kidney specialist may advise a transplant to give you a healthy kidney.

Urinary tract infection

This means infection of the bladder (cystitis), ureters or kidneys (pyelonephritis). Both men and women with diabetes are prone to urinary tract infection (often abbreviated to UTI). The symptoms are frequent burning urination, with cloudy, smelly urine. You may feel generally below par with upset blood glucose control. If the kidneys are infected, there may be a high fever and loin pains; you may feel awful.

Treatment of urinary tract infection

- Drink a pint of water at the first sign of trouble and keep drinking (not alcohol) as much as you can until all the symptoms settle. See your doctor as soon as possible.
- Antibiotics – once a urine specimen has been sent to the laboratory to identify the bacterium causing the infection

your doctor will start antibiotic treatment. Take the full
course of antibiotics, even after you feel better. If you do
not the infection may return.
- Control your blood glucose. Infection increases resistance
to the action of insulin.

Summary

- If you have proteinuria or other signs of diabetic
nephropathy you must pay close attention to risk factors
and have regular kidney checks.
- Keep your blood glucose as close to normal for as much
of the time as possible. Keep to your diabetic diet and
maintain normal weight will help.
- Have your blood pressure checked several times a year.
If it is high work with your doctor to return it to normal
and keep it there.
- Do not smoke.
- Urinary tract infections are common in people with
diabetes, especially women. Treat them promptly – lots
of fluids, see your doctor, provide a sterile urine
specimen for laboratory analysis and take the full course
of antibiotics.
- Everyone with diabetes should have their urine tested
for protein at least once a year.

13

Nerves

Paul is a draughtsman. He has had diabetes for seventeen years, treated by diet and oral hypoglycaemic pills. He works from home and there are always drawings all over the house. One evening in the bath he was horrified to discover a drawing pin embedded in the sole of his right foot, with surrounding redness. Paul could not remember standing on the pin but it must have been there for several days. Even now it did not hurt at all. He pulled out the pin and some pus trickled out of the hole. He cleaned the wound, covered it and went straight to his doctor. Paul had diabetic nerve damage – neuropathy – the soles of both feet had lost all sensation. Paul's foot healed and he has been much more careful ever since.

Diabetic neuropathy

Our nerves are the electric cables which transmit the signals from the brain to all parts of the body. They tell which muscle to move and when. The nerves also convey signals from the body to the brain, relaying information about pain, pressure, temperature, for example. These nerves are called the peripheral nervous system. We also have nerves which monitor our bodily processes like eating, blood pressure, heart rate. This is called the autonomic nervous system. In diabetes both the nerve itself and its fatty sheath can degenerate. The tiny blood vessels supplying the nerves may become blocked. Changes occur in the composition of the nerves, with accumulation of various compounds. All these factors alter the function of the nerve – just like a faulty electric cable. In some instances the wrong signals may be transmitted, in others no signal at all can travel along the nerve.

Risk factors for diabetic neuropathy

High blood pressure

Diabetic neuropathy is notoriously difficult to measure accurately for the purposes of clinical studies. However, several groups have shown that high blood glucose concentrations are associated with worsening of some nerve functions. In people with IDDM, maintaining near-normal blood-glucose concentrations slows the progression of neuropathy (see page 90).

Duration of diabetes

One-quarter to a half of all people with diabetes will have some evidence of neuropathy after twenty years. Again estimates depend on how neuropathy is measured.

Symptoms of diabetic neuropathy

Peripheral neuropathy

- Loss of sensation – this includes numbness, loss of touch, pain, temperature, position, pressure and vibration sensation.
- Altered sensation – 'walking on cotton wool', pins and needles or tingling feelings, irritation.
- Pain – burning or tight pains, mainly in the feet, occasionally occur in neuropathy. Sometimes it is hard to describe the pain, which is due to confused signals being transmitted up the nerve.
- Weakness of a muscle or muscles – this may affect just one small muscle, or several muscles – in the leg, for example, causing limping. Abdominal muscles may even be affected.

Autonomic neuropathy

- Loss of warning of hypoglycaemia.
- Dizziness or faintness on standing, due to postural hypotension.
- Diarrhoea – due to autonomic neuropathy of the bowel.
- Vomiting – due to failure of the stomach to empty.
- Difficulty emptying the bladder.
- Sweating while eating – called gustatory sweating.
- Impotence.

What your doctor may do

First of all, he will want to clarify your symptoms. It is helpful if you know exactly where the numbness is or which movements seem weak; try to work it out before you see your doctor. He will also look for evidence of other causes of neuropathy, like drinking too much alcohol, chemical exposure or vitamin deficiencies. Then he will examine you generally, paying special attention to movements, sensation, coordination and reflexes.

Tests

He will check glucose balance and blood vitamin B_{12} and folate levels. Sometimes neuroelectrophysiological testing is also used. This simply means measuring the tiny electrical impulses that flow down nerves. You may feel little shocks as the nerves are tested but it is rarely an unpleasant procedure.

Peripheral neuropathy

Any peripheral nerve anywhere in the body can be affected by diabetes. The commonest pattern is a 'glove and stocking' sensory loss, the feet being more often affected than the hands. The person may complain of numbness up to his ankles and examination may also find that he has no awareness of vibration or temperature sensation. The level to which each sensory function is lost varies. Vibration sense is often lost first.

Another form of damage is called diabetic amyotrophy.

There is no or little loss of sensation but weakness and wasting of the leg muscles, usually thighs, one side more than the other.

Painful neuropathy is rare. It probably means that the nerves are not dead but partially damaged. There is usually constant burning pains in the feet or legs, sometimes worse at night or in the warmth. The pain may disturb sleep and make walking difficult. It usually settles with time.

Treatment of peripheral neuropathy

Blood glucose control

This can prevent the condition from worsening and in some cases improves it. If the blood glucose is kept within normal limits with insulin therapy some cases of painful neuropathy may improve.

Vigilance

If you have a numb area of skin, take care not to damage it and check every evening at bedtime for rubs or scratches.

Drugs

Painful neuropathy is sometimes helped by amitriptyline, phenytoin or carbamazepine.

Autonomic neuropathy

Loss of warning of hypoglycaemia

The nerves which cause the release of adrenaline (epinephrine) function abnormally and the fear and fast heart beat associated with hypoglycaemia may not be felt. Sweating is not always stopped. This is not the only explanation of loss of warning.

Postural hypotension

A fall in blood pressure on standing is often noted in diabetic clinic measurements, but few of the patients notice any symptoms. Some people become very dizzy when they stand, particularly on getting out of bed in the middle of the night. Usually no specific treatment other than some commonsense is needed. If you get giddy when you stand, rise slowly from your chair and hold on to it until you feel steady enough to move off. When getting out of bed sit on the edge with your feet on the ground for a while, then stand. Stay by the bed until you feel ready to move. If you need to urinate at night sit on the toilet whether you are a man or a woman – it is safer.

Severe postural hypotension may be improved by retraining the body, e.g. elevating the head of the bed so that you sleep on a slight upward slope. Elastic stockings may help when you are standing. Make sure that you do not become dehydrated – in hot weather, for example, or because you have polyuria from a high blood glucose. Fludrocortisone may be used for severe symptoms which do not respond to the other measures.

Diabetic diarrhoea

This is usually watery, sometimes with mucus, and may wake you up early in the morning with the need to rush to the toilet. Beware of postural hypotension at these times. There is rarely any pain but the abdomen may be distended. Because the bowel nerves are not working properly food is hurried along without being properly digested. There may also be other parts of the bowel which become stagnant at times, allowing unusual bacteria to grow. It is important to exclude non-diabetic bowel problems, so your doctor will examine you carefully and may order X-rays of the bowel.

For treatment it is worth a trial of an antibiotic like tetracycline. If this does not work, codeine phosphate usually slows the bowel down. If you have severe diarrhoea you may be fluid- or potassium-depleted, so drink plenty of fruit juice and water.

Diabetic eating problems

Gustatory sweating is fairly common and harmless, although it does have nuisance value. Avoid the foods which make it worse (e.g. spicy foods). If severe, it can be treated with anticholinergic drugs or tiny doses of clonidine. Vomiting due to the stomach not emptying is rare but may make the diabetes hard to control. It may also produce an unpleasant fullness after meals. Metoclopramide or cisapride may help the stomach to empty.

Urinary retention

This is due to a sluggish bladder in neuropathy, but is more often because of prostate enlargement. If you have bladder neuropathy downward pressure on the lower abdomen behind the pubic bone may help you to empty your bladder. Watch for urinary infection (see page 123).

Impotence

Impotence in men with diabetes is usually (as in men without diabetes) temporary. It may be because you have been generally unwell, with uncontrolled diabetes for example. It may be because you are worried about something, like an unhappy love affair, financial problems, depression or trouble at work. The trouble is that the more anxious you become about your sexual performance, the worse it becomes. If you still have wet dreams and morning erections, even if you cannot succeed in intercourse, you are unlikely to have much wrong with the penis or its nerve supply. If you feel generally unwell in any way see your doctor for a full check-up.

Discuss your worries with your partner – it is not fair to keep her in the dark and she will need reassurance that you still care for her. While you are trying to sort things out do not attempt full intercourse; agree that you will give each other pleasure by kissing or caressing only. This removes the anxiety from what is otherwise an enjoyable experience. Most men find that their ability to achieve full intercourse gradually returns.

If you are having no erections at all it is more likely that you have a physical problem with the penis, its nerve or blood supply, or the male sex hormone, testosterone. The other cause of impotence is drugs; this includes those for hypertension – methyl dopa for example – antidepressants and some tranquillisers. Consult your doctor. He will examine you carefully and will check your hormone balance and general physical state. Hormone deficiency is uncommon but is usually easily cured by testosterone injections. If you are not hormone deficient, testosterone is useless – it increases the desire without improving the performance. Occasionally people with atherosclerosis of the pelvic blood vessels have impotence which may be helped by a surgical artery bypass operation.

A few men with diabetes do have impotence due to neuropathy. It is always worth trying the effect of improving blood glucose control, which may help to reduce the nerve damage. Injections can be used to induce erection. Inflatable penile prostheses may be helpful and some centres also use penile implants. Tourniquets are potentially hazardous, though. New devices use a vacuum in a condom-like sheath (Correcaid, ErecAid, Pos-T-Vac). Air is sucked out of the sheath producing the vacuum, drawing the penis to the end of the sheath, and the increasing vacuum induces erection.

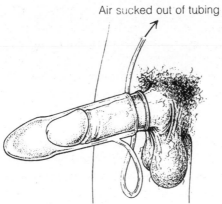

Air sucked out of tubing

Penis drawn gently into device by vacuum

Correctaid™ erection assistance device for impotence. The erection is induced by an increasing vacuum in the sheath.

Nerve entrapment

People with diabetes are more prone than others to trapped nerves. The commonest site is at the wrist, where the median nerve passes through a fibrous tunnel to supply some of the fingers. The bones at the wrist are the carpal bones – hence the name carpal tunnel syndrome. This produces tingling in the fingers and sometimes pain and weakness. The symptoms are often worse at night. The condition is readily treated by slitting the fibrous band which is squashing the nerve.

Summary

- Diabetic neuropathy is an insidious condition. It is common in people who have had diabetes for a long time.
- Symptoms of peripheral neuropathy include loss of sensation or altered sensation, rarely pain, and muscle weakness.
- Symptoms of autonomic neuropathy include loss of warning of hypoglycaemia, postural dizziness, diarrhoea, vomiting, difficulty emptying the bladder, sweating while eating and impotence.
- Report any of these symptoms to your doctor.
- Keep your blood glucose levels within the normal range to prevent neuropathy developing or worsening.
- Be vigilant. Check feet and shoes every day.

14

Skin, joints and feet

The skin in diabetes

Many people do not realise that diabetes can affect the skin, although the problem is rarely serious. Persistent minor skin infections may lead a doctor to test the urine for glucose and hence diagnose diabetes.

Spots and pimples

People with uncontrolled diabetes are prone to spots, boils and carbuncles. Simple spots usually clear as the blood glucose returns to normal. Boils and carbuncles may need draining by a doctor. If you seem very prone to boils try washing in chlorhexidine soap or one of the other proprietary antiseptic soaps. If this fails you may be carrying bacteria in your nose – ask your doctor to send swabs to the laboratory and treat this if indicated.

Thrush

Monilia, candida or thrush are all names for the same fungal infection which grows in damp, sweaty or sugary environments. It is most commonly found in the vagina and perineum of women with diabetes. In this situation it causes a profuse, very itchy, creamy-white discharge and leaves curd-like white deposits on the skin. The perineum may be very red and sore. This is treated by controlling the blood glucose and applying local antifungal cream (miconazole and nystatin for example). The cream must be introduced high into the vagina with the applicator provided, or as a tampon. Men can develop thrush with penile discharge and irritation and the same cream is used. Your partner must always be treated as well. Elderly people, especially if they have been unwell, may develop thrush in their mouths. It is treated with nystatin mouth-wash or amphotericin lozenges. Clean the dentures very carefully. Fat people may develop thrush in skin creases. Antifungal cream will cure it, but the problem will recur if you do not make the creases disappear by losing weight. Complete the full course of antifungal treatment even if the symptoms have gone. There are also single dose antifungal tablets.

Lumps and dents

Repeated injections of insulin into the same area can cause both lumps (insulin hypertrophy) and dents (insulin atrophy). This is caused by reaction of the fatty tissue to insulin. To prevent such lumps and dents rotate your insulin injections so that each area of subcutaneous tissue has as few injections as possible.

When you first start insulin treatment you may develop red spots at injection sites. These are usually transient and the problem settles after a few weeks. If the red spots persist discuss them with your diabetes adviser.

Necrobiosis lipoidica diabeticorum

This is a rare condition in which red patches or dents appear in the skin, usually on the legs. This is harmless and may respond to steroid creams.

The joints in diabetes

Many people with diabetes have minor stiffness of the fingers on careful examination. Others may have tightening of fibrous bands, trapping nerves (see page 131). A very few have more serious joint problems.

Cheiroarthropathy

Despite the name, this is not a serious or sinister problem. Many people with insulin-dependent diabetes develop slight stiffening of the fingers so that they can no longer press them flat against a table. This rarely progresses to anything which needs treatment, but if you have stiff fingers exercise them every day by playing an imaginary or real piano and by flexing and straightening them.

Dupuytren's contracture

This is a tightening of the ligaments and tendons which travel through the palm of the hand to the fingers. If it progresses, the fingers are gradually drawn in and curved. It is thirty times more common in people with diabetes than in non-diabetics. It also occurs in families and in people with liver problems. If it proves a problem a surgeon can release the tendons.

Charcot joints

These are very rare.

Ed had a fast bike that was his pride and joy. One day while kick-starting it the bike kicked back and knocked his ankle. It did not hurt and Ed ignored it. Ed had had diabetes for twenty of his twenty-five years. He never tested his blood or urine and ate what he fancied. He hobbled along to the diabetic clinic some two months after his injury, for which he had not sought help. His ankle was swollen and non-tender – in fact sensation was absent below the knee. On X-ray the ankle joint was destroyed. This was a Charcot joint, created by walking on a badly-injured but painless ankle and by the circulatory problems of diabetes. Poor Ed died a year later from kidney failure after a lifetime of neglected diabetes.

Feet in diabetes

Foot problems are one of the commonest reasons for admission to hospital of people over forty who have diabetes. As many as one in six people with diabetes have foot ulcers at some time in their diabetic career.

Risk factors with feet

Dirt and sweat

You should wash your feet as often as you wash your face. This means washing them every day with soap and rinsing well with warm water. Dry them carefully, especially between the toes. Change your socks, stockings or tights every day and more often in hot weather.

Ill-fitting shoes

Ever since the shoe became an attractive item of clothing and not just a foot protector, the foot has been vulnerable to the whims of fashion. A good shoe should have a moderate heel, be shaped so that the foot does not slide around when you walk (lace-ups are best from this point of view), have a comfortable toe which does not squeeze your toes either from the sides or above, and above all should feel comfortable the first time you put it on. Never buy shoes which have to be 'broken in'. If your shoes start to hurt take them off immediately, and if you cannot make them completely comfortable stop wearing them.

Pebbles in your shoes

In tropical countries explorers always check their boots for snakes before putting them on in the morning. People with diabetes need to be equally wary of stones, loose linings, cracks in the shoe, nails or any unevenness that may rub your skin.

Faulty toenail cutting

Cut your toenails straight across and never leave sharp points or edges. Never cut the nails in a curve as this will cause ingrowing toenails. Your nails will be easiest to cut after a bath, but do not cut them too short. Use purpose-made toenail clippers if you have difficulty with scissors. If the nails are very thick or you cannot cut them yourself ask a chiropodist to do it. Never allow your nails to grow too long or to dig into other toes.

Do-it-yourself corn care

Don't! Never attempt to cut out your own corns and do not use corn plasters. See a chiropodist.

Garters

Some older people prefer garters to suspender belts for stockings. Garters constrict the circulation and should not be worn.

Hard dry skin

If you have any areas of hard dry skin look to see if your shoes are rubbing. Rub away the hard skin after your bath (never cut it) and use foot cream (hand cream will do) to keep the skin supple. Do not let the skin get so dry that it cracks, but, equally, do not put so much cream on that the feet go soggy.

Walking barefoot

This is not a good idea as the feet get very hard, dirty and are easily cut or bruised. If you have neuropathy you are at special risk. Shoes were invented to protect the feet – wear them.

Athletes' foot

This condition looks like soggy blisters, usually between the toes. Other infections may get into the bloodstream through cracks in the athletes' foot. Your doctor will give you some cream and/or powder, or you can buy it. Use it according to instructions, even if all signs of athletes' foot have gone. If you are particularly prone to athletes' foot some chiropodists suggest regular use of surgical spirit on the feet to prevent reinfection. This will also tend to harden the feet. Wash your bath mat regularly.

Diabetic neuropathy

Because this reduces pain, temperature and touch sensation, people with neuropathy are at greater risk of injuring themselves than others and the injury may go undetected for longer. A small rub which would lead a non-neuropath to change his shoes may carry on for days if you have neuropathy. Or a hot-water bottle may burn, unknown to you. A well-maintained electric blanket used according to instructions is better. If you injure your foot, infection may get in and become severe before it is treated because the pain this would normally produce is blunted.

If you know you have neuropathy look at your feet every night for rubs or other injuries when you wash them. Use a mirror if you cannot bend over.

Diabetic arterial disease

Atherosclerosis in the arteries of the leg will reduce the amount of blood circulating in the feet. This means that the tissues heal more slowly and are more vulnerable to cold. The smaller vessels in the feet may also be affected and the circulation damaged further. Signs of poor circulation are intermittent claudication (see page 105), loss of hair on the lower leg, cold feet and slow colour change when you press on the skin and release it or when you elevate and then lower the foot.

If you have poor circulation keep your feet warm in winter – I have seen frostbite in two Oxford men with diabetes. Warm socks and shoes or boots (e.g. lined with sheepskin) are helpful. Pay attention to the risk factors on pages 85–89. Stop smoking.

Arthropathy

This is rarely considered. However, if you can develop cheiroarthropathy (page 135), the same applies to the toes. Stiff toes may assume clawed positions and be more at risk of rubbing on the shoes. Make sure your shoes do not squash your toes from above or from the sides. Keep your toes wiggling!

Chiropody and podiatry

Everyone with diabetes should have a chiropodist or podiatrist. If you have perfect feet your chiropodist will help you to keep them that way. If you have foot problems he or she will help sort them out and prevent them from recurring. You should see your chiropodist at regular intervals. It is especially important for you to attend a chiropodist if you are stiff or have visual problems and find caring for your feet difficult. Ideally you should be able to telephone your chiropodist at any time for an urgent appointment if you have an acute foot problem.

Foot ulcers

These are responsible for many months of hospital admission for a few people with diabetes. They develop from tiny wounds which become infected or are in a place which keeps getting knocked or rubbed. They gradually enlarge and become chronically infected. They may become deeper and there may be surrounding soft-tissue infection (cellulitis) or deeper abscesses. Rarely the infection may become so severe that the person's life is at risk and the limb has to be amputated.

This all sounds horrifying but it is important to remember that ulcers can be prevented by proper foot care. If you notice anything wrong with your feet – a cut, graze, discoloured area or blister – you should report it to your doctor, nurse or chiropodist immediately. If skin is broken clean it straightaway with sterile cotton wool or gauze, and clean water. Dry it with sterile gauze and cover it with a non-stick sterile dressing (e.g. N-A Dressing) kept on with a bandage. Avoid adhesive tape if possible and use light 'non-allergy' tape if necessary. This dressing will keep it clean. Clean and dress the wound every day as advised by your doctor until it is completely healed. Avoid proprietary antiseptics unless advised by your doctor as they can cause skin irritation in people with skin allergies. Try to find out why you injured your foot so that you can prevent it from happening again. If your injury has been caused by, or is worsened by, rubbing of your shoes, protect it from further rubbing and stop wearing those shoes. Rings of chiropody felt around an injury can take the pressure off it – your chiropodist will advise you.

Established ulcers take longer to treat. They should be cleaned and dressed every day (twice a day for very sticky ones) by someone who knows what he or she is doing. This can be you or your relatives, providing you have been taught exactly what to do by an expert. All the slough in the bottom must be thoroughly cleaned out until nothing but healthy tissue remains (if this hurts take a painkiller first). If there is cellulitis, antibiotic treatment will be needed. Abscesses need surgical drainage. The ulcer must not be knocked or rubbed while it is healing. This means that if it is on the sole of the foot or touches your shoes you should not walk on it until it is well healed. This may mean bed rest, a weight-bearing plaster or special shoe. It is much better to take the time to heal the ulcer properly. Do not be tempted to walk on it.

The infection may upset your blood glucose control. Check your blood glucose four times a day and adjust your treatment with your diabetes adviser's help to ensure that your blood glucose remains normal.

Special shoes

If you have neuropathy, pressure areas on your feet, arthritic or misshapen toes, bunions, or have had previous foot ulcers, you may benefit from special shoes and insoles to protect your feet. These shoes can be made to measure and are designed to take the pressure off at-risk areas and be completely comfortable all over.

Summary

- Minor skin and ligament problems are common in diabetes, but rarely troublesome.
- Look after your skin. Bad boils or skin infections and thrush require the attention of your doctor and will settle rapidly with treatment.
- Dents and lumps can appear after repeated insulin injections in the same site. Rotate your insulin injection sites.
- Keep your joints supple.
- If you have numb feet, remember that even serious injuries may not hurt. People with diabetes must look after their feet. See your doctor if you damage yourself.
- Wash your feet every day and dry them well, checking for cracks or injuries.
- Contact your doctor, nurse, chiropodist or podiatrist immediately if you notice anything wrong with your feet.
- Choose your shoes carefully. They should fit comfortably from the moment you buy them. Examine them before you put them on (remember the snakes!) Wear clean socks, stockings or tights every day. Wear special shoes if necessary.
- Cut your toenails straight across, with no rough edges. Ask your chiropodist to cut them for you if it is difficult.
- See your chiropodist or podiatrist regularly.

15

Caring for older people

This chapter is written mainly for people who are caring for an older relative or friend with diabetes. There are increasing numbers of people with a half-century of diabetes behind them who are well and active in their seventies, eighties or nineties. However, some people who have had diabetes for forty or fifty years may have to contend with problems of diabetic tissue damage as well as those of growing older. New diabetes is also common in older people. Overall the prevalence of diabetes in elderly people is about 8 per cent.

Diagnosis

The symptoms of diabetes may be less obvious in an elderly person than in someone young. Older people do not always have severe thirst or polyuria but may just appear vaguely unwell or listless; they may gradually lose weight, despite apparently eating normally. Elderly persons with diabetes may take longer to recover from viral or bacterial infections. Diabetes may be diagnosed because of tissue damage following many months or years of unnoticed hyperglycaemia. Testing the urine for glucose is simple and quick and should be part of the routine examination of all elderly people who are unwell.

Treatment

Diet

'You can't teach an old dog new tricks.' Not wholly correct, but this saying has some truth in it. A person may find it hard to alter the diet that they have enjoyed for seventy years. Do not attempt to introduce an entirely new diet all at once. The first step should be a change from sugar in tea, puddings and so on to the use of artificial sweeteners. Avoid other sugar-containing foods; substitute plain high-fibre biscuits for sugary ones. Then after a few weeks add small amounts of bran to cereals and puddings. Try putting beans into casseroles. Buy or make lentil soup occasionally. Work towards phasing out the white bread and replacing it with wholemeal.

Too much fibre may produce indigestion and wind in someone usually on a low-residue diet, so go gently. It may take six months to alter all the components of the diet so that the older person is eating a 'diabetic diet'. It is better to be patient than to have meals refused or total rejection of the recommended diet.

Oral hypoglycaemic pills

Of people whose diabetes is diagnosed over the age of sixty, 80 or 90 per cent can be treated successfully without insulin. This is obviously easier for all concerned when caring for older people, but should not deter a doctor from giving insulin to a patient who really needs it, whatever the difficulties. Furthermore, at time of illness insulin may need to be used temporarily.

Some elderly people have hazy memories and may not remember to take their medication – or may forget that they have taken it and take an extra dose. There are several 'organiser' pill boxes available but if you cannot buy one, make one – for example, using a small cardboard or plastic box. Fill the box daily or weekly as required. Make sure that the pills can be got out of the box easily, though.

There is some debate as to which oral hypoglycaemic pills are best for older people. As you grow older the body may be less efficient at breaking down drugs and clearing them from the body. Very long-acting drugs like chlorpropamide, and medium- to long-acting drugs like glibenclamide may take several days to clear from the body. This means that an episode of hypoglycaemia may last for hours or days or recur after treatment with food or glucose. It is important to remember that oral hypoglycaemic drugs probably increase the amount of insulin released from the pancreas in response to food. Thus, food given to treat a hypoglycaemic episode may cause further insulin release and 'rebound hypo-glycaemia'. The remedy is to keep a close check on blood-glucose levels and keep giving food and glucose. In Britain we tend to use short-acting sulphonylurea drugs which can be given in small, divided doses; for example, tolbutamide or glipizide. It is never a good idea to take a sulphonylurea before bed unless you are specifically told to do so by a physician.

The older you are the more medicines you are likely to be taking. These drugs may interact with each other or may cause alterations in glucose tolerance. As an elderly person may be seeing several clinics or doctors it is vital that every doctor seen is shown the total medication list.

An elderly person should always carry a list which includes:

- current and previous illnesses, and operations;
- current *pills, medicines, injections*, skin or eye treatments;
- *drugs* to which he/she is *allergic*;
- he/she should show these lists to *every* doctor he/she sees, every time he/she sees them, especially in the emergency department.

Insulin treatment

Many elderly people give their own insulin injections and adjust the dose as necessary. Insulin pens may be easier to handle than syringe/needle and insulin bottle. However, some elderly people have problems with vision, dexterity and comprehension. Visual problems such as cataracts or diabetic retinopathy may make it very hard to see the tiny lines on the insulin syringe. There are several devices which may overcome this. Some allow the syringe to preset at the correct amount (e.g. BD Cornwall syringe, Dos-Aid, Insul-gage). Click-count syringes give an audible click every two units – but if you are taking a lot of insulin you may lose count of the clicks. A large magnifying glass fixed to a table or shelf may help to show up the divisions on the syringe and any air bubbles. There are magnifying devices which fit on to the syringe (C-Better, Char-Mag, Magni-Guide, Syringe Magnifier). Some devices fix the bottle or emphasise the top so that it is easier to guide the needle into the bung (Holdease, Inject-Aid, Injection Safety Guard, Insulin Aid, Insulin Needle Guide). These may also help people with stiff fingers from arthritis, problems with coordination or shakiness.

Some elderly people cannot draw up their own insulin but can still inject it. In this case a nurse or family member can draw up a day's or week's supply to be kept in the refrigerator or in a commercial or home-made pre-drawn syringe case. Make sure that morning and evening doses are clearly identified if different. This is also one way of ensuring that the elderly person remembers whether or not the insulin has been given – if the full syringe is still there it has not! Pens with visible insulin cartridges are helpful for people who sometimes forget that they have given themselves their insulin; checking off on a chart is another method. However, if someone is very forgetful, a friend, nurse or relative has to inject the insulin once or twice a day to make certain that it has been given.

Stiff limbs and joints may reduce the number of injection sites which can be reached by an elderly person. They can usually manage to inject into thighs or abdomen but the twisting needed for injections into the buttock may be impossible and injections in the arms may also be difficult. Again, if a person is unable to manage their injection because of physical disabilities someone else will have to do it.

The insulin regimen requires some thought. If an elderly person finds any aspect of drawing up or giving insulin difficult they should have the simplest effective insulin regimen possible. Once-daily insulin is simpler than twice daily but may not always provide such good blood-glucose control. Very long-acting insulin – Ultratard, for example – provides background activity for twenty-four hours and can be used with a single shot of fast-acting insulin in some people. However, it takes several days to clear from the body.

IF FOUND - PLEASE RETURN TO OWNER AS SOON AS POSSIBLE. THANK YOU.

D I A B E T I C   M E D I C A L   C A R D

NAME Elizabeth Star

ADDRESS 31 Sky Appartments, 22 East Moon Street, Sunnyville

PHONE NO. 012 345 6789

EMERGENCY CONTACT Mrs Flower/012 543 9876

DOCTOR Dr Tree, Leaf Green Surgery, Sunnyville 098 765 4321

CURRENT MEDICATIONS

Betaxolol Eye Drops 0.25%
Insulin: Isophane 12 units
  (before breakfast)
  Isophane 8 units
  (before evening meal)

MAJOR ILLNESS & OPERATIONS

1931 TB   1982 Glaucoma
1943 Hysterectomy   1985 Diabetes
1965 (R) hip replacement

ALLERGIES   Aspirin, Penicillin

A card like this should be carried and shown to every doctor you see, every time you see them, especially in emergency departments.

If an elderly person has a night-time hypoglycaemic attack – after unexpected exercise or a missed meal, for example – she may be hypoglycaemic for a long time because the insulin does not 'wear off' for many hours. On the other hand, very fast-acting insulin given before a meal which is delayed for some reason or forgotten altogether may produce rapid severe hypoglycaemia, even though the insulin will wear off more quickly. A fixed proportion mixture – for example 30 per cent rapid acting with 70 per cent medium acting – removes the need for separate drawing up and mixing. There are now several such mixtures on the market which provide good blood-glucose balance in people whose meals and exercise are similar each day. They will probably need to be given twice a day.

No single insulin regimen is right for everyone – the insulin must be tailored to each person's needs.

Glucose monitoring

Urine-glucose testing

The easiest form of glucose monitoring is with urine testing strips (see pages 21–22). The strip can be held in the urine stream and read at the appropriate time by most normally-sighted elderly people. While this does give a general idea of what is happening, and is probably better than not testing at all, the kidney threshold for glucose excretion is often high in older people. This means that by the time glucose appears in the urine the blood glucose may be well above normal. If the kidney threshold is known, urine tests can still be helpful and are certainly simpler than blood tests.

The results should be recorded in a diabetic diary and you should know at what level to call for help. Discuss this with the diabetes adviser. A rough guide is to ask the doctor or nurse for help if the urine glucose is 2 per cent or more for three days, or over 1 per cent for a week. Seek help immediately if the elderly person feels ill. Persistently negative urine tests may indicate that the insulin or oral hypoglycaemic pills could be reduced.

Blind people can check their own urine glucose using a meter which gives audible bleeps for each glucose level.

Blood-glucose testing

This is the best guide to what is happening but is a waste of time and effort unless it is done properly. With the current enthusiasm for blood-glucose monitoring, many elderly people are taught how to do this, and some spend many miserable hours trying to obtain results which are inaccurate and which they do not understand.

Susan is sixty-five years old. She has had insulin-treated diabetes for ten years. Two years ago she was shown how to measure her blood glucose and has been bringing her carefully-recorded results to clinic ever since. They were always below 10 mmol/l (180 mg/dl).

A new doctor surprised Susan one day by asking her to show him how she measured her glucose. She pricked her finger, smeared some blood on to a piece of cotton wool, peered at the red smudge and announced that her blood glucose was 6 mmol/l (108 mg/dl)!

Agatha is seventy-three. She was shown how to measure her blood glucose level and given a diary in which to record the results. At her next clinic visit she triumphantly produced her diary. Each page was covered in neatly placed spots of congealed blood! Agatha had forgotten that she was meant to put the blood on the test strips, not in the diary itself.

It is important that everyone who is blood-glucose monitoring checks their technique from time to time (this includes doctors and nurses). If an elderly person cannot check their own blood glucose then someone else should do it for them – a relative, friend or nurse. It should be checked at least once a week and more often if unwell or anything unusual happens. Four measurements on one day each week would be even more helpful, but may be harder to organise.

And what blood glucose concentration should an elderly person with diabetes have? We should be aiming for normal blood glucose levels in everyone with diabetes regardless of age. However, people with normal blood-glucose levels are more likely to become hypoglycaemic than those with higher blood-glucose concentrations.

A young person can usually recognise and treat a hypoglycaemic attack more rapidly than an elderly person. A young person's body is also more able to withstand the changes in the circulation which occur during hypoglycaemia. In particular, hypoglycaemia can cause changes in the blood flow to the brain, and elderly people's stiff arteries may not be able to cope with this readily. An elderly person living alone may fall or become unconscious during a hypoglycaemic attack.

A low blood-glucose level prevents shivering and hypoglycaemic people can therefore become hypothermic. Elderly people are already at risk of hypothermia because they are less able to keep warm in cold weather than youngsters. A compromise, balancing prevention of tissue damage and of hypoglycaemia, seems best, although every elderly diabetic person's treatment should be adjusted individually.

I usually suggest that the blood glucose is kept between 6 and 10 mmol/l (108 and 180 mg/dl). I would not worry unduly about the occasional 13 mmol/l (234 mg/dl). I would, however, worry if the blood glucose was always over 10 mmol/l (requiring an increase in hypoglycaemic therapy or exercise or a reduction in diet). I would also want to know about any hypoglycaemic attacks or blood-glucose levels below 4 mmol/l (72 mg/dl). Discuss the blood-glucose level you should be aiming for with the diabetes adviser and ask at what level to contact him or her. As a rough guide, call for help if the blood glucose is over 20 mmol/l (360 mg/dl) for three days (seek help immediately if the elderly person feels or looks ill), if he or she has any hypoglycaemic attacks or a blood glucose below 4 mmol/l (72 mg/dl), and if the blood glucose is above 10 mmol/l for a week.

Hyperglycaemia

High glucose levels cause general realise, lack of energy and thinking problems. However, some elderly people can tolerate extremely high blood-glucose levels with few complaints. Frequent trips to the toilet or urinary incontinence (see page 154) and obvious thirst are clues. They will gradually lose weight. Old people can easily become short of fluid (dehydrated) which may make them tired, lethargic or confused. They may not be able to drink enough to keep up with the urinary fluid loss. Also if someone usually has a glucose level of, say 20 mmol/l (360 mg/dl), a minor viral infection can easily increase that to 30 mmol/l (540 mg/dl), producing severe dehydration, major disturbances in blood chemistry and coma. Thus it is important to keep a regular check on the blood glucose and to act early if it is raised.

Once you have become used to adjusting insulin or pill treatment you will be able to sort out minor glucose fluctuations yourself. Try to learn the clues that show you that the elderly person you care for is in diabetic difficulties. Call for help early rather than later.

Hypoglycaemia

Many older people have the same warnings of hypoglycaemia as young people. However, the intensity of the warning can lessen as people age, or the symptoms may change. Older people are more likely to be on older medication such as beta blockers (page 98) which modify the warning symptoms. Just as in the young, the blood-glucose concentration at which symptoms appear varies from person to person. Some older people may feel very unwell with blood-glucose levels between 3 and 4 mmol/l (54 and 72 mg/dl). Others may tolerate blood glucose levels of 2 mmol/l (36 mg/dl) without complaint.

It is nearly always possible for an observer to see some clue of the onset of a hypoglycaemic attack in someone they know well. This may be confusion or forgetfulness – indeed such symptoms in someone with diabetes should always make one think of hypoglycaemia. It may be slight pallor or sweatiness, irritability or 'cussedness' or considerable slowness of response. The problem can be spotting a change in someone who is always a little muddled or who always looks pale. Have a high index of suspicion – check the blood glucose if you are worried. If you cannot measure the blood glucose give some sugar or glucose and note what happens. Glucose gel in polythene squeeze bottles (Hypostop or Glutose) can be particularly useful.

A forgetful old person may not eat their meal or may neglect to cook it at all so keep a check on the larder. Unaccustomed exercise – a special outing or a household emergency – may precipitate a hypoglycaemic attack. Sunny weather may also do so by tempting an elderly person out to do some gardening.

In cold weather it is very important to remember the dual dangers of hypoglycaemia and hypothermia. Hypothermia is commoner in people with diabetes than non-diabetics. If you can, invite your elderly relative or friend to stay until the weather is better.

Thinking

We all think slightly more slowly as we grow older. Someone with atherosclerosis in the arteries supplying the brain may have more difficulty in thinking things through and remembering. It is often the most recent events which are forgotten first. This can be very irritating for a carer who has to repeat the same story many times or search for lost clothing, spectacles or books. Writing things down may help. Remember that it is very frustrating to find that your thoughts are muddled or your memory poor, so try to remain sympathetic. And remember that confusion and forgetfulness can signal hypoglycaemia.

Bert is eighty-four and has had chlorpropamide-treated diabetes for two years. Home urine tests were always negative. He lived alone. He had influenza and for some weeks afterwards felt unwell and had no appetite. He became muddled, forgetting what day it was and sometimes not recognising his family. One night the neighbours found him wandering in the road in his pyjamas.

He was admitted to hospital where he was found to be thin, cold and dirty. He had no idea where he was or even who he was. His blood glucose was 2 mmol/l (36 mg/dl). A glucose injection somewhat improved his thinking and after twenty-four hours of glucose infusions into a vein he was able to converse normally. In retrospect he had probably been hypoglycaemic for much of the few weeks prior to his admission because he had eaten very little following his influenza. He went to live with his daughter and his blood glucose was controlled on a small dose of tolbutamide.

Diabetes is common in people with some forms of dementia, e.g. those associated with multiple small strokes, of whom 20 per cent are diabetic. Thinking ability (cognitive function) is reduced if the blood glucose is persistently high. Studies have shown that diabetes in people with severe memory problems or dementia may not be cared for as vigorously as in someone who has all their faculties. But poor diabetes care can worsen the dementia and cause the patient much misery. It can also make carers' jobs much harder.

Body maintenance

Eyes

Many older people need to wear spectacles because the shape of the eye changes with age. Cataracts can occur in anyone but are more common in diabetics (see pages 115, 171). They are treatable. Nowadays there are increasing numbers of people who have had diabetes for over fifty years. Some of them have tissue damage, including retinopathy, although many are remarkably free from complications of diabetes. Tissue damage can be prevented and treated in people of all ages.

Someone with diabetes should *never* ignore changes in their vision as 'just old age' but should always seek an immediate eye check. Blurred vision is also a sign of glaucoma – raised pressure inside the eye; this is also treatable and is more common in diabetics. One of the commonest causes of blurred vision in diabetes is high blood-glucose levels, so check these and act to improve the glucose control if necessary (see page 112). Even if you suspect that the blurring is simply poor glucose balance, always ask an expert to check the elderly person's eyes. And never let them buy new glasses until the ophthalmologist says the eyes are stable – they may just waste their money.

One in three elderly people with diabetes have visual problems. One in ten newly diagnosed people with diabetes will already have retinopathy.

Feet

In Chapter 14 I described how diabetes can affect the feet. This is especially important in older diabetics. Foot ulcers are one of the commonest reasons for admission of elderly diabetics to hospital. Once an ulcer has developed it may take months or even years to heal. An old person should check his or her feet every single day. A mirror and a table light may help them to see the bits that they cannot reach.

If the elderly person is too stiff to reach their feet they should be encouraged to ask someone else to look. Danger areas are numb or tingly patches, bunions or clawed toes, and areas of hard skin on the sole of the foot. If they do have pressure areas or distorted or numb feet there are several types of specially made-to-measure shoes and insoles.

If they have poor circulation they must keep their feet warm in winter. Firm, wool- or fur-lined boots or shoes may help. Loose slippers, apparently so comfortable around the house, are dangerous and proper shoes are better, even indoors.

Washing and hygiene

It is important to keep every part of the body clean as small cracks in the skin may allow bacteria to enter the system and cause major infection. Dirt and loose skin may also rub and cause sore places. Everyone tries their best to keep clean but if the elderly person has arthritis or other physical problems they may not be able to reach some parts. Places like skin creases and the navel tend to get missed; between the toes is another difficult place to reach. The elderly person may need help with washing.

There are many shower and bath aids and in Britain some of these may be provided by the state. Similarly, rails and other supports are available. It is worth enquiring.

The skin may become very dry because there is less fatty tissue in it, so keep it supple with a bland cream or oil. It is better to rub the oil into the skin after the bath than to pour it into the bathwater, which makes the bath very slippery.

Urinary incontinence

One obvious reason for incontinence in diabetes is a high blood-glucose, causing polyuria. If someone is immobile they may not reach the lavatory in time. Nocturnal incontinence may be due to a moderately long-acting once-daily insulin wearing off allowing the glucose to rise. Urinary tract infections (page 123) are common in older women and diabetics – you may notice an unpleasant fishy smell. The infection causes irritability of the bladder and an urgent desire to pass urine. Again the urine may leak out before the lavatory is reached. A course of antibiotics can work wonders. Other local causes such as prolapsed vagina or urethral problems may cause incontinence. Prostate disease is the commonest cause of incontinence in men. A stroke may reduce mobility or alter pelvic sensations or bladder function. Faecal constipation is a common treatable cause of urinary incontinence. Diuretic medication (pages 102 and 123) can induce urinary urgency, while drugs which make an older person sleepy, confused or dizzy can reduce awareness of the need to pass urine or slow the journey to the lavatory. Other forms of confusion may reduce awareness of urination.

Urinary incontinence is thus a common problem so there is no need for the elderly person to be embarrassed. They should be encouraged to seek help – a full medical examination is essential to find the cause of the incontinence. While the cause is being identified and treated, stick-on sanitary pads are available for minor leakages and larger incontinence pads and pants can be used if necessary, while there are penile sheaths for men. The doctor, health visitor or nurse will be able to provide these or they can be bought in the chemists or drugstores. Protect the mattress and chairs with plastic sheeting. There are also disposable sheets or bed padding, and state laundry services may be able to help. There are urinals for both men and women, or a commode can be placed in the bedroom or close at hand. Regular urination, whether or not the elderly person feels the need to pass water, may reduce the number of leaks.

Bowels

Constipation can be one of the features of high blood glucose – the polyuria causing dehydration and excess absorption of fluid from the gut. Plenty of fluids and control of the blood glucose will usually resolve the problem. In contrast, diabetic autonomic neuropathy can cause diarrhoea. However, this is uncommon and diarrhoea is much more likely to be caused by overflow in someone who is constipated, overuse of laxatives or gastroenteritis. A change in bowel habit should be reported to the doctor.

Getting about

Numb feet, foot ulcers, balance problems, arthritis or a stroke may make getting about rather difficult. Falls are frightening and may break bones. Postural hypotension (page 128) is quite common in older people, not just because of diabetic autonomic neuropathy, but also because of medication taken to lower blood pressure for example.

A stick may provide all the support that is needed, but for more disabled people a walking frame can be very helpful. Diabetic neuropathy may feel like walking on cotton wool or may destroy the positional sense in the feet. Something to lean on is comforting in this case.

The elderly person may need help transferring from bed to chair or chair to lavatory. Higher, firm chairs are easier to get out of and the height of the bed can be adjusted. A saggy bed is difficult to get on and off. The greatest risk of postural hypotension is at night, when getting up to urinate. Slow rising and a commode by the bed helps.

Immobility

If someone has had a stroke or has other disabilities they may be unable to move themselves. A few people with diabetes have amputations of legs or feet. This in itself should not cause immobility as artificial limbs can be provided. However, combined with other disabilities, it may reduce mobility.

If you are caring for an immobile person it is vital that their skin is protected. Bedsores or pressure sores in a diabetic can take months to heal and may cause blood poisoning, not to mention major suffering. The areas to watch are the lower back and buttocks, the heels and any bony prominences. Sheepskin or artificial purpose-made padding under all areas at risk, careful washing, drying and oiling of the skin with frequent turning can all prevent bedsores. Special mattresses, e.g. ripple or water mattresses, can also be used. If your relative becomes immobile discuss prevention of bedsores with the nurse and doctor immediately – it can happen overnight.

You also need to prevent joints and muscles becoming stiff or contracted. Learn how to lift and turn your relative without injuring them or you. Find out all you can about aids and allowances. Caring for someone who is severely disabled is hard work and an expert job. It can certainly be done very well at home and be very rewarding, but do make sure you learn exactly what to do from the experts and do not take on more than you can handle. Very few people with diabetes become severely immobile.

Diabetes care is important

Elderly people or their carers may gain the impression that diabetes is a mild condition and that other illnesses that the person has are more important. Some elderly people with diabetes (about 7 per cent) receive no professional diabetes care at all. They are more likely to die than those receiving care. Specific diabetes care can either be within general practice or a hospital diabetes clinic or a combination of the two. Make sure your elderly person gets the best that is available locally.

Many conditions other than diabetes are worsened or more difficult to treat in a diabetic person. For example, a heart attack may be more severe or an infection take longer to resolve. Diabetes complications such as high or low glucose emergencies (or comas) are harder to treat in the elderly, so particular care should be taken to prevent them. Overall elderly people with diabetes, when compared with non-diabetic people of the same age, see their general practitioners more, need more hospital care, have a higher rate of prescribing for conditions other than diabetes and need more help in the home.

Remember to tell every health professional that the elderly person has diabetes and make sure you know how to get expert diabetes help when it is needed.

The carer

Many people care for elderly relatives or friends. You share common problems with them but have the additional responsibility of caring for diabetes. This means that you need to know as much about diabetes as any diabetic. Try to ensure that you always attend clinic or medical consultations with your relative (if they agree). Make a list of questions and concerns. Learn all you can about diabetes; this book should help, while others in the series are *Diabetes: The Complete Guide* and *Diabetes: A Beyond Basics Guide* by Rowan Hillson. *Caring for an Elderly Relative* by Keith Thompson will also help you. But above all, remember to look after yourself too. If you need assistance ask for it.

Summary

- Most elderly people with diabetes are fit and well and care for themselves.
- A few older diabetics need help from carers.

- Diagnosis of diabetes in the elderly may rely on subtle symptoms and signs and can be delayed. Diabetic tissue damage may be present at diagnosis.
- Adjust the diet gently. Do not introduce too much fibre too early in someone unused to it. Eventually aim for a full diabetic diet.
- Most elderly people can be treated with diet alone or with diet and oral hypoglycaemic pills. The type of pill should be chosen carefully to suit the patient's lifestyle and to avoid hypoglycaemia.
- Insulin treatment should also be tailored to the diabetic person's needs.
- Balance the risks of hyperglycaemia with the risks of hypoglycaemia. Hypoglycaemia is more hazardous in the elderly than in young people.
- Hyperglycaemic elderly people may not report symptoms. Frequent urination, occasional incontinence and thirst, with weight loss and perhaps constipation are clues. Beware of dehydration.
- Hypoglycaemia may not cause classic symptoms. Confusion can warn of hypoglycaemia in the elderly.
- Any change in vision should be reported to the doctor – it is rarely 'just old age'.
- Feet are especially vulnerable. Protect them.
- Unsteadiness or difficulty walking can be helped with a stick or walking aid. Do not let pride come before a fall.
- If you are caring for an immobile elderly diabetic person protect their skin, especially pressure areas. Learn how to care for them from the experts and find out all you can about aids and allowances.
- If you are caring for an elderly person and his or her diabetes, learn all you can about diabetes. It will improve their life and reduce your worry.

16

Everyday life

Organisation of diabetes care

Self care

As soon as possible get into a routine of diabetes care. Become practised at blood-testing and pill- or insulin-taking. Soon it will become as much a part of your daily routine as washing or shaving. Remember to check for signs of tissue damage.

Carry glucose

Always carry glucose on your person if you are taking oral hypoglycaemic pills or insulin. This can be in the form of glucose tablets, Hypostop, sweets or candies. Keep emergency glucose under your pillow or by your bed at night.

Carry a diabetic card

Always carry a diabetic card. These can be obtained from your national diabetes association or your clinic. Until you have a standard card, make yourself one stating:

I AM DIABETIC
If I am found ill or fainting, please give me sugar.
If I do not respond, please call a doctor.
My name is . . .
Address . . .
In an emergency contact . . .
My diabetes treatment is . . .

Some cards have international messages – see illustration.

Warning tags

Medic-Alert and other organisations provide warning med-allions or bracelets and some keep more detailed records, e.g. SOS. You may feel that this is helpful.

Your diabetes adviser

Be clear about who your professional adviser is. This will vary, depending on where you live. In America or Australia you may have a private diabetes specialist or diabetologist who is solely responsible for your diabetes care. In Britain

DIABETIC DIABETIC

I AM DIABETIC

JE SUIS DIABÉTIQUE

ICH BIN DIABETIKER

મને મીઠા પેશાબની બીમારી છે.

مجھے ذیابیطیس (شوگر) کی بیماری ہے

मैं पेशाब में शूगर का/की मरीज़ हूं ।

मैं भ्रुगर दा/दी मरीज़ हां ।

আমি একজন ডায়বেটিক রোগী ।

I AM A DIABETIC
If I am found ill or fainting:

● Please give me some sugar
  (about 2 tablespoons)
  – either in water
  – or as sugar lumps
  –or as sweets
    (I may be carrying these)

● If I fail to recover
  – call a doctor
  – or an ambulance to take me to
    hospital

A card like this should be carried and shown to every doctor you see, every time you see them, especially in emergency departments.

you may also have a private diabetologist, although most people tend to remain within the National Health Service. This means that your general health will be cared for by your general practitioner (GP) who may also care for your diabetes. Other GPs will refer you to a hospital diabetologist.

Whoever you see, it is important that your condition is reviewed regularly (at least once a year and preferably more often) by someone who is experienced in the care of people with diabetes. This review should encompass assessment of your recent blood glucose control and general examination for signs of tissue damage. It is also an opportunity for you to learn more about your diabetes and to ask any questions you may have.

Establish who to contact for emergency help before you need it and which telephone number to call.

The diabetes care team

Nowadays many centres have a team of people working together to care for you and your diabetes. This may include specialist diabetes nurses, educators, dietitians, chiropodists and secretarial and clerical staff. In some areas there is a liaison officer who is usually trained in nursing and can provide help between the hospital and your home. She or he may be especially helpful in the first few days at home as a new diabetic. Many liaison officers or diabetes specialist nurses will give you emergency telephone numbers and come out to help you if you are in difficulties with your diabetes.

The system

Every medical care facility has a system. You will have to communicate with your health care team for many years so learn the system now. Many diabetics attend a clinic in a large hospital under the care of a particular consultant or specialist. Find out his name. He will have varying numbers of doctors responsible to him – they are called interns and residents in America and house officers, senior house officers, registrars and senior registrars in Britain. Much of your care will be carried out by these younger doctors. However, if you particularly want to see your specialist or consultant in person do ask – this can always be arranged.

Clinic appointments are usually made via an appointments clerk. She may organise bookings for a lot of different clinics so you must know which clinic (e.g. Dr Sweet's tuesday morning diabetic clinic) you belong to. It is usually more reliable to alter clinic appointments by writing to the appointments officer (ascertain the exact address from the person concerned). Telephone messages can get lost easily in busy offices.

It helps to put your hospital record number on all correspondence. Your hospital records will be kept by a records department supervised by a records officer. Diabetes records are kept separately in some centres. If you change your name (e.g. get married) or your address or your GP, please let your specialist know and also send a copy to the hospital medical records officer. If you attend another clinic in the same hospital, for example the varicose veins clinic, always tell the doctors there that you have diabetes and attend the diabetic clinic, and vice versa at the diabetes clinic.

The clinic visit may take longer than you anticipate so go prepared by taking a book and a snack. Most clinics run appointment systems but much can happen to disrupt these. For example, the doctor may have to deal with an emergency in the clinic or elsewhere in the hospital. Your doctor will probably want to examine you so please wear clothes that are easy to take off and put back on. You will certainly be asked about your home blood- or urine-glucose monitoring and your current medication so bring records of this with you (see page 146). Some diabetic clinics see fifty to one hundred people each session. All the staff will be working hard, so please be patient. However, if you feel that you have waited unduly long please remind the receptionist or clinic nurse that you are still waiting. If you have constructive suggestions about the clinic please tell the doctor.

Join your national diabetes association

There are diabetes associations all over the world. Most of them are national bodies with local groups. They exist not only to support people with diabetes but to further research into diabetes and to act as a national voice to improve diabetes care. They produce journals for people with diabetes and for health care professionals, and other information of all kinds. It is well worth joining your national and local groups, if only to learn about current facilities and new advances in diabetes care. Some people with diabetes find that talking with other diabetics is comforting and also allows sharing of new ideas and techniques to make life more comfortable or flexible. The addresses of some national diabetes associations are given at the end of the book.

You local clinic may also have a diabetes group.

Driving

Most people with diabetes can drive, but you must comply with the law. In Britain you must report your diabetes to the Driver and Vehicle Licensing Authority (DVLA) and to your motor insurance company. If you are treated with insulin injections your licence will be renewed every three years, subject to a satisfactory medical report. The licence is usually only withheld if you have had recurrent hypoglycaemic attacks or if you have a form of diabetic tissue damage which makes it impossible for you to drive safely (e.g. poor vision). If you are taking oral hypoglycaemic pills you will be granted a standard licence valid until age 70. If your diabetes can be controlled by diet there is no need to inform the DVLA of your condition. If there is a change in your general medical condition, you should of course, inform them.

Never drive when you are hypoglycaemic, and take care to avoid becoming hypoglycaemic whilst driving. For example, eat a snack before driving home in the evening. Carry food and canned or boxed soft drinks in the car.

Drivers of large goods vehicles (LGV) and passenger carrying vehicles (PCV) may face some restrictions. In the

UK, people on insulin treatment are not allowed to drive passenger vehicles, but most of those on oral hypoglycaemic pills can hold both PCV and LGV licences, provided there are no other contraindications. LGV licences are considered individually in insulin-treated drivers. If you have problems, phone the BDA Careline on 0171 636 6112.

Full details are available in a BDA Patient Information Booklet entitled *Driving and Diabetes* (BDA, 1996).

Insurance

You should tell your insurance companies that you have diabetes and what treatment you are taking for this. This may cause them to increase their premiums, although some companies give better rates than others to people with diabetes. Obtain several quotations and also seek advice from your diabetes association. Remember that the other healthy aspects of your life such as being a non-smoker, within your ideal weight and taking regular exercise may reduce your rate with some companies. Full details are given in a BDA Patient Information Booklet entitled *Insurance and Diabetes* (BDA, 1996), or phone their Careline on 0171 636 6112.

In Britain people who have passed the Advanced Driving Test can obtain reduced motor insurance premiums. Consider taking the test and becoming a member of the Institute of Advanced Motoring.

Work

Having diabetes should not interfere with your work. Unless your contract stipulates it, you are under no obligation to reveal your diabetes to your employer. However, it is usually best to be open and honest about your diabetes. If you drive a company vehicle or operate machinery you *must* tell your employer you have diabetes – your diabetes doctor can write a supportive letter if necessary.

If you take oral hypoglycaemic pills or have insulin injections it is sensible to discuss your diabetes with your colleagues at work, as they will then be able to help you in the unlikely event of a hypoglycaemic episode. People with insulin-treated diabetes should not risk hypoglycaemia because they lack the courage to ask for time to eat a mid-morning or mid-afternoon snack – it is always possible to arrange this. Keep some biscuits or candy bars at work for emergencies and find somewhere clean to do blood-glucose tests. You may need to take extra food to work if you cannot predict your workload, so that you can eat more to cover periods of increased exertion.

If you are applying for a new job, most prospective employers ask about health or require a medical examination. It is foolish to conceal your diabetes as this may render your contract void. If you can demonstrate that you are fit and have full and confident control over your diabetes it should not reduce your employment prospects.

Holidays

Diabetes is no bar to a wonderful holiday, in your own country or abroad. When travelling make sure that you have enough food and soft drinks to cover the journey and delays, duplicate bottles of insulin or pills, syringes and needles if necessary, your glucose testing kit, your diabetes card (including a note in the language of the country you are visiting) and emergency glucose. It is important to take out adequate travel insurance.

For more advice about work and travel read *Diabetes: A Beyond Basics Guide*, by Rowan Hillson, in this series.

Family

When you tell your family that you have diabetes it will obviously be as much of a shock for them as it was for you. However they should also be relieved that the problem has been diagnosed and that treatment is possible – they may have been worrying about you for some time. Explain that having diabetes will not stop you from taking a full part in all aspects of family life and that you will be able to carry on with your work and your hobbies. When someone we love is ill, we all want to help, so do not shut your family out. Encourage your close family to learn about diabetes with you, to learn how to check your blood glucose and to give you your insulin. Learn about the diabetic diet as a family – it is a healthy diet for anyone to follow. After a while your diabetes will simply be a part of you, accepted by the family but no 'big deal'.

Never allow your diabetes to take up too large a part of your life or that of your family – occasionally, wives or husbands become over-obsessional about diabetes.

Enjoy life

There is no need for diabetes to overshadow everything else; quite the reverse, give it a little matter-of-fact commonsense care each day along the guidelines given to you by your diabetes care team and this book, and spend the majority of your time doing whatever you want in life.

Remember: you control your diabetes – it does not control you.

Now go out and enjoy life to the full.

GLOSSARY

acidosis   Condition in which blood is more acid than normal.
adipose tissue   Body fat.
adrenaline   (American name **epinephrine**) 'Flight, fright and fight' hormone produced by the adrenal gland under stress.
angina   Chest pain caused by insufficient blood supply to heart muscle (a form of ischaemic heart disease). Also known as angina pectoris.
angiogram   X-ray examination of an artery.
ankle oedema   Swelling of the ankles.
aorta   The largest artery in the body, running from the heart through the chest and abdomen. The aorta carries blood from the heart for distribution into other arteries around the body.
arteriopathy   Abnormality of artery.
artery   Vessel which carries blood from the heart to other parts of the body.
arthropathy   Abnormality of joint.
atherosclerosis   Hardening and furring up of the arteries.
autonomic nervous system   Nerves controlling largely automatic body functions such as heart beat, blood pressure and bowel movement.
autonomic neuropathy   Abnormality of the nerves controlling body functions.
background retinopathy   The common form of diabetic retinopathy with microaneurysms, dot-and-blot haemorrhages and exudates.
balanitis   Inflammation of the penis.
beta blocker   Drugs which reduce high blood pressure, steady the heart and prevent angina. All the names end in -olol, e.g. atenolol.
biguanide   A type of blood-glucose lowering pill.
blood pressure   BP. Pressure at which blood circulates in the arteries.
carbohydrate   CHO. Sugary or starchy food which is digested in the gut to produce simple sugars like glucose. Carbohydrate foods include candy or sweets, cakes, biscuits, soda pop, bread, rice, pasta, oats, beans, lentils.
cardiac   To do with the heart.
cardiac enzymes   Chemicals released by damaged heart muscle.
cardiac failure   Reduced functioning of the heart causing shortness of breath or ankle swelling.
carotid angiogram   X-ray of dye passing up the carotid arteries into the brain arteries.
carotid artery   One of two arteries which run one each side of

the neck to supply the head and brain.
cataract Lens opacity.
cells The tiny building blocks from which the human body is made. Cell constituents are contained in a membrane.
cerebral embolus Clot from another part of the body which lodges in an artery supplying the brain.
cerebral haemorrhage Bleeding into the brain.
cerebral infarct Death of brain tissue due to insufficient blood supply.
cerebral thrombosis Clot in an artery supplying the brain.
cerebrovascular disease Disease of the arteries supplying the brain.
Charcot joints Damaged joints in areas of neuropathy (rare).
cheiroarthropathy Stiffening of the hands.
chiropodist Someone who prevents and treats foot disorders.
chiropody Treatment and prevention of foot disorders.
cholesterol A fat which circulates in the blood and is obtained from animal fats in food.
computerised tomogram CT scan. X-ray which can take multiple, very detailed films from different angles. Commonly used to look at the brain, but whole-body CT scanners are also available.
congestive cardiac failure Impaired pumping of the right ventricle of the heart causing ankle swelling.
conjunctivitis Inflammation of the conjunctiva (membrane covering the white of the eye and inner eyelid).
continuous ambulatory peritoneal dialysis CAPD. An out-patient system of filtering wastes from the body of someone in kidney failure. Clean fluid is run into the abdominal cavity, takes up the waste substances and is run out again.
continuous subcutaneous insulin infusion CSII. A system for the constant pumping of insulin through a fine needle left under the skin all the time. Also known as an insulin pump.
coronary artery Artery which supplies the heart muscle.
coronary thrombosis Clot in an artery supplying heart muscle.
creatinine Waste chemical produced by breakdown of protein in the body and passed through the kidneys into the urine. A measure of kidney function.
cystitis Inflammation of the urinary bladder.
diabetes insipidus Condition in which large volumes of insipid urine are passed, due to lack of anti-diuretic hormone.
diabetes mellitus Condition in which the blood glucose concentration is above normal, causing passage of large amounts (diabetes – a siphon) of sweet urine (mellitus – sweet, like honey).
diabetic amyotrophy A form of diabetic nerve damage

which causes weak muscles, usually in the legs.

dialysis Artificial filtration of fluid and waste products which are normally excreted in the urine by the kidneys.

diastolic blood pressure Blood pressure between the heart beats.

diet What you eat.

dietitian Someone who promotes a healthy diet and advises on dietary treatments.

diuretic Pill which increases urinary fluid loss. Diuretics are used to treat cardiac failure and most are also effective blood-pressure lowering drugs.

dot-and-blot haemorrhage Tiny bleeds into the retina in diabetic retinopathy.

Dupuytren's contracture Tightening of the ligaments in the palm of the hand or fingers.

dysphasia Difficulty in talking.

dysuria Pain or discomfort on passing urine.

echocardiography Examination of heart using ultrasound waves from a probe run over skin of chest.

electrocardiogram ECG or EKG. Recording of electrical activity of heart muscle as it contracts and relaxes.

electrolytes Blood chemicals such as sodium and potassium.

enzyme Body chemical which facilitates other chemical processes.

epinephrine See adrenaline.

essential hypertension High blood pressure for which no specific cause can be found.

fat Greasy or oily substance. Fatty foods include butter, margarine, cheese, cooking oil, fried foods.

femoral arteriogram X-ray of dye injected into a femoral artery.

femoral artery The main artery supplying each leg. The femoral pulse can be felt in the groin.

fibre Roughage in food. Found in beans, lentils, peas, bran, wholemeal flour, potatoes, etc.

fluoroscein angiogram Photographs of fluoroscein dye passing through the blood vessels in the eye.

gastroenteritis Inflammation or infection of the stomach and intestines; a tummy bug.

gastrointestinal To do with the stomach and intestines.

glaucoma Raised pressure inside the eye.

glomeruli Tangles of tiny blood vessels in the kidneys from which urine filters into the urinary drainage system.

glucose A simple sugar obtained from carbohydrates in food. Glucose circulates in the bloodstream and is one of the body's main energy sources.

glucose tolerance The body's ability to process glucose.

glycaemia Glucose in the blood.

glycogen   The form in which glucose is stored in liver and muscles.
glycosuria   Glucose in the urine.
glycosylated haemoglobin   See haemoglobin Al$_c$.
guar gum   A substance which slows the absorption of carbohydrate from the gut.
gustatory sweating   Sweating while eating.
haemodialysis   Artificial filtration of blood in someone with kidney failure.
haemoglobin Al$_c$ Haemoglobin (oxygen-carrying chemical in red blood cells) to which glucose has become attached. A long-term measure of blood glucose concentration.
haemorrhage   Bleed.
heart   Muscular organ which pumps blood around the body.
heart attack   General non-specific term for myocardial infarction or coronary thrombosis.
hormone   A chemical made in one part of the body and acting in another part of the body.
hyper-   High, above normal.
hyperglycaemia   High blood-glucose concentration (i.e. above normal).
hypertension   High blood pressure.
hypo-   Low, below normal.
hypoglycaemia   Low blood-glucose concentration (i.e. below normal).
hypotension   Low blood pressure.
hypothermia   Low body temperature.
impotence   Difficulty in obtaining or maintaining a penile erection.
infarction   Condition in which a body tissue dies from lack of blood supply – irreversible.
insulin   A hormone produced in cells of the islets of Langerhans in the pancreas. Essential for the entry of glucose into the body's cells.
insulin-dependent diabetes   IDDM. See Type I diabetes.
insulin receptor   Site on the cell surface where insulin acts.
intermittent claudication   The intermittent limping caused by insufficient blood supply to the leg muscles.
intravenous urogram   X-ray of the kidneys showing the excretion of dye injected into a vein.
ischaemia   Condition in which a body tissue has insufficient blood supply – reversible.
ischaemic heart disease   An illness in which the blood supply to the heart muscle is insufficient.
islet cells   Cells which produce insulin.
islets of Langerhans   Clusters of cells in the pancreas. One form of islet cells produces insulin.

juvenile-onset diabetes Diabetes starting in youth. IDDM. Type I diabetes.

ketoacidosis A state of severe insulin-deficiency causing fat breakdown, ketone formation and acidification of the blood.

ketones Fat breakdown products which smell of acetone or pear-drops and make the blood acid.

kilocalories Cals or kcals. A measure of energy, for example in food or used up in exercise.

kilojoules Another measure of energy. One kilocalorie = 4.2 kilojoules.

left ventricle Chamber of the heart which pumps oxygenated blood into the aorta.

left ventricular failure Reduced functioning of the left pumping chamber of the heart causing fluid to build up in the lungs and shortness of breath.

lens The part of the eye responsible for focusing (like the lens of a camera).

lipid General name for fats found in the body.

liver Large organ in upper right abdomen which acts as an energy store, chemical factory and detoxifying unit, and which produces bile.

macroangiopathy Disease of large blood vessels such as those supplying the legs.

macrovascular disease Macroangiopathy.

macula Area of best vision in the eye.

macular oedema Swelling of the macula.

maturity-onset diabetes Diabetes starting over the age of thirty. This term usually implies that the person is not completely insulin deficient, at least initially. Non-insulin-dependent diabetes. Type II diabetes.

metabolism Chemical processing of substances in the body.

microalbuminuria The presence of tiny quantities of protein in the urine.

microaneurysm Tiny blow-out in the wall of a capillary in the retina of the eye.

microangiopathy Disease of small blood vessels such as those supplying the eyes or kidney.

myocardial infarction Death of heart muscle caused by lack of blood supply.

myocardium Heart muscle.

necrobiosis lipoidica diabeticorum Diabetic skin lesion (rare).

nephropathy Abnormality of the kidney.

nerve Cable carrying signals to or from the brain and spinal cord.

neuroelectrophysiology Study of the way nerves work.

neuropathy Abnormality of the nerves.

nocturia Passing urine at night.

non-insulin-dependent diabetes NIDDM. Diabetes in which insulin treatment is not essential initially. See Type II diabetes.
obese Overweight, fat.
obesity Condition of being overweight or fat.
oedema Swelling.
ophthalmoscope Magnifying glass and torch with which the doctor looks into your eyes.
oral Taken by mouth.
-pathy Disease, abnormality, e.g. neuropathy, retinopathy.
palpitations Awareness of irregular or abnormally fast heart beat.
pancreas Abdominal gland producing digestive enzymes, insulin and other hormones.
paraesthesia Pins and needles or tingling.
peripheral nervous system Nerves supplying the muscles attached to the skeleton and registering body sensation such as touch, pain, temperature.
peripheral neuropathy Abnormality of peripheral nerves, e.g. those supplying arms or legs.
peripheral vascular disease Abnormality of blood vessels supplying arms or legs.
photocoagulation Light treatment of retinopathy.
polydipsia Drinking large volumes of fluid.
polyunsaturated fats Fats containing vegetable oils such as sunflower seed oil.
polyuria Passing large volumes of urine frequently.
postural hypotension Fall in blood pressure on standing.
protein Dietary constituent required for body growth and repair.
proteinuria Protein in the urine.
pruritus vulvae Itching of the vulva or perineum.
pyelonephritis Kidney infection.
receptor Site on the cell wall with which a chemical or hormone links.
renal To do with the kidney.
renal glycosuria The presence of glucose in the urine because of an abnormally low renal threshold for glucose.
renal threshold Blood glucose concentration above which glucose overflows into the urine.
retina Light-sensitive tissue at the back of the eye.
retinopathy Abnormality of the retina.
right ventricle Chamber of the heart which pumps the blood from the body into the lungs to be oxygenated.
right ventricular failure Reduced functioning of the right pumping chamber of the heart causing fluid to build up in the legs and ankle swelling.
risk factor A factor which makes you more likely to develop

a particular problem than someone who does not have this factor.

saturated fats   Animal fats, e.g. those in dairy products, meat.

stroke   Abnormality of brain function (e.g. weakness of arm or leg) due to disease of the arteries supplying the brain or damage to the brain.

subcutaneous   Under the skin.

subcutaneous fat   The fatty tissues under the skin.

sulphonylurea   A form of blood-glucose lowering pill.

systolic blood pressure   Pumping pressure of the heart, as measured in the arteries.

testosterone   Male sex hormone.

thrombosis   Clotting of blood.

thrombus   A blood clot.

thrush   Candidiasis or moniliasis. Fungal infection caused by Candida albicans fungus. Produces white creamy patches and intense itching and soreness.

transient ischaemic attack   TIA. Short-lived stroke with full recovery within twenty-four hours.

triglyceride   Form of fat which circulates in bloodstream.

Type I diabetes   Diabetes due to complete insulin deficiency for which treatment with insulin is essential. Lack of insulin leads to rapid illness and ketone production. Juvenile-onset diabetes. Insulin-dependent diabetes. IDDM.

Type II diabetes   Diabetes due to inefficiency of insulin action or relative insulin deficiency, which can usually be managed without insulin injections, at least initially. Ketone formation is less likely. Maturity-onset diabetes. Non-insulin-dependent diabetes. NIDDM.

ulcer   Open sore.

ultrasound scan   Scan of part of the body using sound waves.

uraemia   High blood-urea concentration.

urea   Blood chemical; waste substance excreted in urine.

ureter   Tube from the kidney to the urinary bladder.

urethra   Tube from the urinary bladder to the outside.

urinary incontinence   Unintentional leakage of urine.

urinary retention   Retention of urine in the bladder because it cannot be passed.

urinary tract infection   UTI. Infection of urine drainage system.

visual acuity   Sharpness of vision.

vitreous   Clear jelly in the eye between retina and lens.

vitreous haemorrhage   Bleeding into the vitreous.

USEFUL ADDRESSES

United Kingdom

**Action on Smoking and
Health (ASH)**
109 Gloucester Place
London W1H 4EJ
0171–935–3519

Age Concern
Astral House
1268 London Road
Norbury
London SW16 4ER
0181–679–8000

**British Diabetic
Association**
10 Queen Anne Street
London W1M 0BD
0171–323–1531

**British Sports Association
for the Disabled**
Maryglen Haig Suite
Solecast House
13–27 Brunswick Place
London N1 6DX
0171–490–4919

**Disability Information
Trust**
Mary Marlborough Centre
Nuffield Orthopaedic
Centre
Headington
Oxford OX3 7LD
01865 227592

**Eye Care Information
Service**
PO Box 3957
London SE1 6D7
0171–357–7730

Genesis Medical
7 Heathgate Place
Agincourt Rd
London NW3 2NU
0171–284–2824

**Health Education
Authority**
Mabledon Place
London WC1H 9TX
0171–383–3833

Help the Aged
16–18 St James Walk
London EC1R 0BE
0171–253–0253

Keep Fit Association
Francis House
Francis Street
London SW1P 1DE
0171–233–8898

Medic-Alert Foundation
12 Bridge Wharf
156 Caledonian Road
London N1 9UU
0171–833–3034

Osbon Medical (Erecaid)
29 Pattison Road
London NW2 2HL
0171–431–7003

Partially Sighted Society
Queens Road
Doncaster
South Yorkshire
DN1 2NX
01302–323–132

Ramblers Association
1–5 Wandsworth Road
London SW8 2XX
0171–582–6878

Royal National Institute for the Blind
224 Great Portland Street
London W1N 6AA
0171–388–1266

Royal Association for Disability and Rehabilitation
12 City Forum
250 City Road
London EC1V 8AF

Royal National Institute for the Deaf
105 Gower Street
London WC1E 6AH
0171–387–8033
Minicom 0171–383–3154

The Sports Council
16 Upper Woburn Place
London WC1H OQP
0171–388–1277

Australia

Diabetes Association of SA Inc
157 Burbridge Road
Hilton
SA 5Q33

Diabetic Association of WA
48 Wickham Street
East Perth
WA 6004

Diabetes Australia
5/7 Phipps Place
Deakin
ACT 2600

Diabetes Australia
65 Davey Street
Hobart
Tas 7000

Diabetes Australia (NSW)
149 Pitt Road
Redfern
NSW

Diabetes Australia (Queensland)
124 Gerler Road
Hendra
QLD 4011

Diabetes Education and Assessment Centre
74 Herbert Street
St Leonards
NSW 2065

Diabetes Foundation (Vic)
100 Collins Street
Melbourne
Vic 3000

Diabetes Research Foundation of WA
Queen Elizabeth II Medical Centre
Hollywood
Perth
WA 6000

Canada
The Canadian Diabetes Association
(National Office)
15 Toronto Street
Toronto
Suite 1001
Ontario M5C 2EB

United States
American Diabetes Association
National Service Center
PO Box 25757
1660 Duke Street
Alexandria
VA 22314

Independent Living Aids Inc
1500 New Horizon Boulevard
Amityville
NY 11701

Juvenile Diabetes Foundation International
432 Park Avenue South
New York
NY 10016

National Association for the Visually Handicapped
22 West 21st
New York
NY 10010

National Diabetes Information Clearing House
Box NDIC
Bethesda
MD 20892

SOURCES OF INFORMATION

C.S. Cockram, T. Dutton and P.H. Sonkson, 'Driving and diabetes', *Diabetic Medicine*, 3:137–140, 1986.

J.K. Davidson, *Clinical Diabetes Mellitus: A Problem Orientated Approach*, Thieme Inc, New York, 1986.

R.M. Hillson, T.D.R. Hockaday and D.J. Newton, 'Hyperinsulinaemia is associated with development of electrocardiographic abnormalities in diabetics', *Diabetes Research*, 1:143–149, 1984.

R.M. Hillson, T.D.R. Hockaday and D.J. Newton, 'Hyperglycaemia is one correlate of deterioration in vibration sense during the five years after diagnosis of type II (non-insulin dependent) diabetes', *Diabetologia*, 26:122–126, 1984.

R.M. Hillson, T.D.R. Hockaday, D.J. Newton and B. Pim, 'Delayed diagnosis of non-insulin-dependent diabetes is associated with greater metabolic and clinical abnormality', *Diabetic Medicine*, 2:383–386, 1985.

J. Howard Williams, R.M. Hillson, A. Bron, P. Awdry, J.I. Mann and T.D.R. Hockaday, 'Retinopathy is associated with higher glycaemia in maturity onset type diabetes', *Diabetologia*, 27:198–202, 1984.

H. Keen and J. Jarrett, *Complications of Diabetes*, second edition, Edward Arnold, London, 1982.

L.P. Krall (ed.), *World Book of Diabetes in Practice, Volume 2*, B.V. (Biomedical Division), Oxford, 1986.

E. Kritzinger and K. Taylor, *Diabetic Eye Disease*, MTP Press, Lancaster, Boston, 1984.

J.I. Mann, K. Pyorala and A. Teuscher, *Diabetes in Epidemiological Perspective*, Churchill Livingstone, London, 1983.

J.A. Muir Gray and H. McKenzie, *Take Care of Your Elderly Relative*, Unwin Paperbacks, London, 1980.

National Diabetes Data Group, 'Diabetes in America (Diabetes Data compiled 1984)', *National Institutes of Health Publication* No. 85–1468, August 1985.

Royal College of Physicians, 'Obesity', *Journal of the Royal College of Physicians of London*, 17(1):5–65, 1983.

Royal Society of Medicine, 'Biguanide therapy today', *International Congress and Symposium Series*, No. 48, RSM, London; Academic Press Inc. (London) Ltd; 1981.

Royal Society of Medicine, 'Non-insulin dependent diabetes, its present and future'. *International Congress and Symposium Series* No. 68, RSM and OUP, 1984.

The Diabetes Control and Complications Trial Research Group, 'The effect of intensive treatment of diabetes on the development and progression of long-term complications in IDDM.' *New England Journal of Medicine*, 329:977–81, 1993.

A.W. Thorburn, J.C. Brand and A.S. Truswell, 'Salt and the glycaemic response', *British Medical Journal*, 292:1697–1699, 1986.

D.J. Weatherall, J.G.G. Ledingham and D.A. Warrell (eds), *Oxford Textbook of Medicine*, OUP, Oxford, 1987.

INDEX

To order any of these books direct from Vermilion (p+p free), use the form below or call our credit-card hotline on **01279 427203**.

Please send me

...... copies of **DIABETES: THE COMPLETE GUIDE** @ £8.99 each

...... copies of **DIABETES: A BEYOND BASICS GUIDE**
@ £9.99 each

Mr/Ms/Mrs/Miss/Other (Block Letters)

....

Address...

....

....

Postcode................................Signed...

HOW TO PAY

☐ I enclose a cheque/postal order for £................................
made payable to 'Vermilion'

☐ I wish to pay by Access/Visa card (delete where
appropriate)

Card Number ☐☐☐☐☐☐☐☐☐☐☐☐☐☐☐☐☐

Expiry Date ☐☐☐☐

Post order to **Murlyn Services Ltd, PO Box 50, Harlow, Essex CM17 0DZ.**

POSTAGE AND PACKING ARE FREE. Offer open in Great Britain including Northern Ireland. Books should arrive less than 28 days after we receive your order; they are subject to availability at time of ordering. If not entirely satisfied return in the same packaging and condition as received with a covering letter within 7 days. Vermilion books are available from all good booksellers.